CARNICOPIA
The Meat-Based Cookbook
Your Doctor Doesn't Want You to Read

By Cary Kelly

Copyright © 2024 by Cary Kelly

All rights reserved. No part of this publication may be reproduced, distributed, or transmitted in any form or by any means, including photocopying, recording, or other electronic or mechanical methods, without the prior written permission of the publisher, except in the case of brief quotations embodied in critical reviews and certain other noncommercial uses permitted by copyright law.

Library of Congress Cataloging-in-Publication Data
Names: Kelly, Cary, author.
Title: Carnicopia: The Meat-Based Cookbook Your Doctor Doesn't Want You to Read / Cary Kelly.
Subjects: LCHF Carnivore diet. | Cooking (Meat) | Health.
ISBN: 9798344598666

Disclaimer: Personal Experience, Not Medical Advice
The views expressed in this book are solely those of the author based on personal experiences and are not intended as medical advice. Always consult with a healthcare professional before starting any new diet or exercise program.

Design and layout: Sara Hohly
Self-published via KDP

Acknowledgments

This endeavor of creating this cookbook would not have been possible without all my fans on X who encourage and inspire me to continue to create new recipes, and my friend, Sara Hohly, for her dedication and help with design, copy writing, and editing. I'm very grateful for her time and efforts.

Don't blame the candles,
blame the cake.

Contents

Preface vii

Meats 2

Poultry 30

Seafoods 36

Eggs 44

Cheese 50

Extras 58

Desserts 74

Index 81

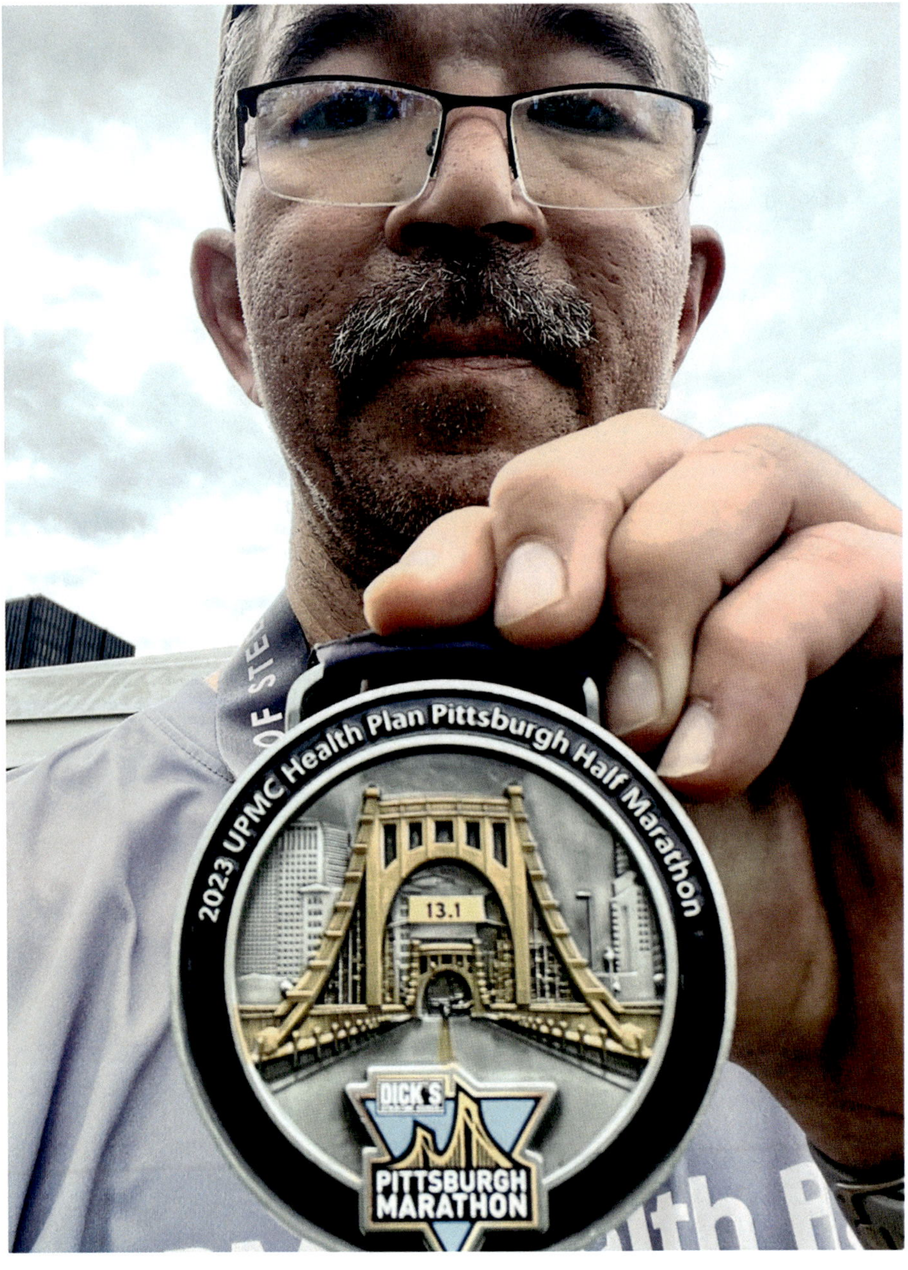
2023 UPMC Health Plan Pittsburgh Half Marathon
13.1
DICK'S
PITTSBURGH
MARATHON

Preface

Welcome to "Carnicopia." Here you'll discover the transformative power of a meat-based diet. It's a path less traveled beyond mainstream interventions, but it's one that has revolutionized my health and vitality.

On September 13, 2018, tipping the scales at over 210 pounds and struggling with depression, inflammation, and exhaustion, I discovered I was likely type II diabetic. This turned out to be a blessing in disguise, as I could have had a heart attack, liver disease, or cancer as a wake up call. In an effort to reclaim my health I embarked on a ketogenic diet. This pivotal decision marked the beginning of my profound transformation. By March of 2019, six months in, I had lost substantial weight and achieved a healthier physique; I realized then the immense impact of dietary choices on my overall well-being.

I transitioned to a carnivore diet in 2020, prioritizing animal products and virtually eliminating carbohydrates. This shift led to further physical improvements, such as significant muscle gains and a stable, healthy weight. These dietary changes also dramatically enhanced my athletic activities. Five years ago I couldn't even run 50 yards. In 2021 I started running, completing my first marathon in 2022, and several half-marathons since then.

In the past 2070 days, I have consumed an estimated 150 pounds of butter, 6000 eggs, and approximately 4200 pounds of red meat. Every bite I take contradicts the mainstream narrative that animal foods are bad for us. Not only am I not dead, I feel better and more alive than ever. There's no such thing as eating a little bit of everything to be healthy. It's really all about eating real nutritious food that has sustained us for generations, namely animal proteins and fats.

I've written this book to advocate for a return to nutrient-rich animal foods. "Carnicopia" is not just a cookbook; it's a manifesto for health. It aims to challenge common misconceptions about dietary nutrients, like the healthiness of plants and vegetable oils, and to call into question the dangers of cholesterol and red meat. I share my evolving collection of delicious animal-based recipes. These dishes have been created to support and encourage a high-protein, low-carb lifestyle, without being too restrictive or monotonous.

Join me in rethinking conventional health-wisdom and embracing a lifestyle that could dramatically change your health. Let's embark on this journey together, to prove that sometimes the best remedy is on your plate and not in your medicine cabinet.

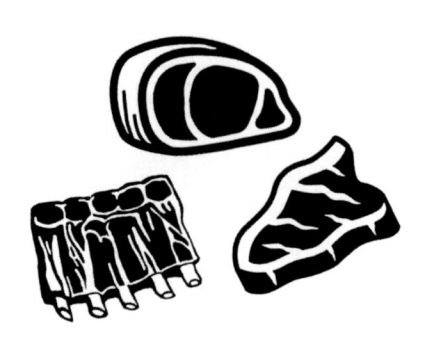

Meat Dishes

Dry Brining

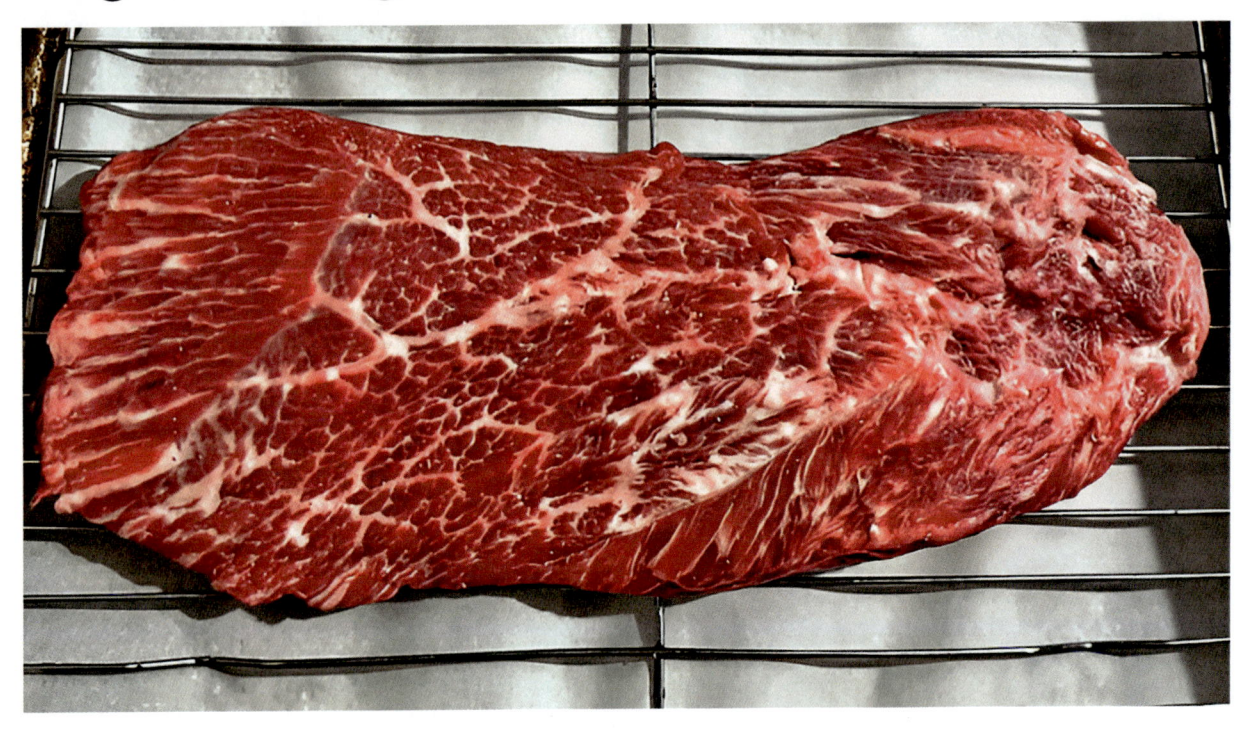

Brining is a technique that uses a salt solution to season raw foods. Traditional brining is done by soaking ingredients in brine which often leads to unsatisfactory and watery results, including a lack of browning. Dry brining on the other hand, works with the natural juices of the meat to create a concentrated brine on the surface, which then gets absorbed back into the meat, enriching the flavor. As the salt diffuses into the meat, it re-shapes and dissolves the muscle proteins, allowing the meat to become tender and retain moisture when it's cooked. The surface of the meat is also much drier than before salting, which allows for much faster browning. The overall results are tender, deeply seasoned, and juicy meats with no loss of flavor. This process is a game-changer for giving beef greater flavor and peak tenderness with minimal effort.

97% of first time dry briners are blown away by the tenderness, flavor and juiciness that this method produces. The 3% who said their dry brining experience was a disaster, used too much salt.

INGREDIENTS

kosher salt, like Maldon, Diamond Crystal, or Morton
meat, such as beef, bison, elk, pork, chicken, or fish
rack and tray set up, to allow air to circulate

TIME

In general at least 12 hours and up to 3 days for large roasts and whole birds. Steaks, chops, and fish fillets can brine for as little as 45 minutes (or up to 24 hours). As a rough guide, allow one day per inch of thickness for best results.

DIRECTIONS

Pat meat dry, lightly salt all sides, edges, and crevices of the meat. The amount of salt to use for dry-brining is correlated to the size of the meat. Sprinkle the salt from several inches above, letting it scatter. Seasoning evenly, with a light dusting is key. Place meat on a rack fitted into a tray, so air can circulate all around it. Refrigerate uncovered for 1 day per inch of thickness, up to 3 or 4 days absolute max.

Notes: If salt is still visible on the meat surface after 24 hours, then there is too much salt. (Be sure to brush off the excess before cooking.) While dry-brining works for all kinds of meat and fish, it's not recommended for ground meats, because they will lose moisture and become dry.

A trick for crispy chicken or turkey skin: mix up ½ cup kosher salt with 2 tablespoons of baking powder for dry-brining. Or for a smaller portion, use 1 teaspoon of baking powder with 1 tablespoon of kosher salt. The baking powder changes the pH of the skin and creates tiny air bubbles for serious crispy crunchiness.

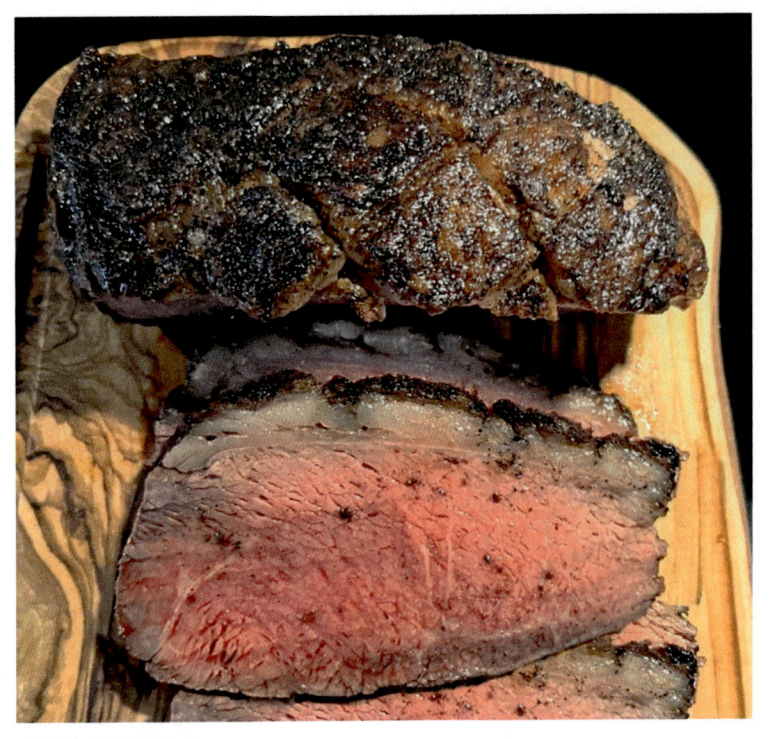

Picanha Roast

This Brazilian sirloin roast with the fat cap is poor man's prime rib. It's also called culotte or top cap sirloin.

CARB COUNT: 0

INGREDIENTS

2-3 pound picanha roast
(top sirloin or culotte with fat cap)
fresh rosemary sprig
4 tablespoons butter
SPOG blend which is equal parts:
salt
paprika
onion powder
garlic power
plus chili powder here

DIRECTIONS

Score the fat cap with a cross hatch (diamond pattern) and then rub and salt the entire roast generously. Pan sear in a skillet with a half stick of butter, browning all the sides. Add the fresh rosemary to the pan to flavor the butter.

Transfer meat to a grated rack and roast at 350°F for about 15 minutes per pound, or until 125°F for medium rare. This should take about 30-45 minutes. Allow 20 minutes for meat to rest. Scrape up leftover butter and spices from the pan into a ramekin and use as a tasty dipping sauce.

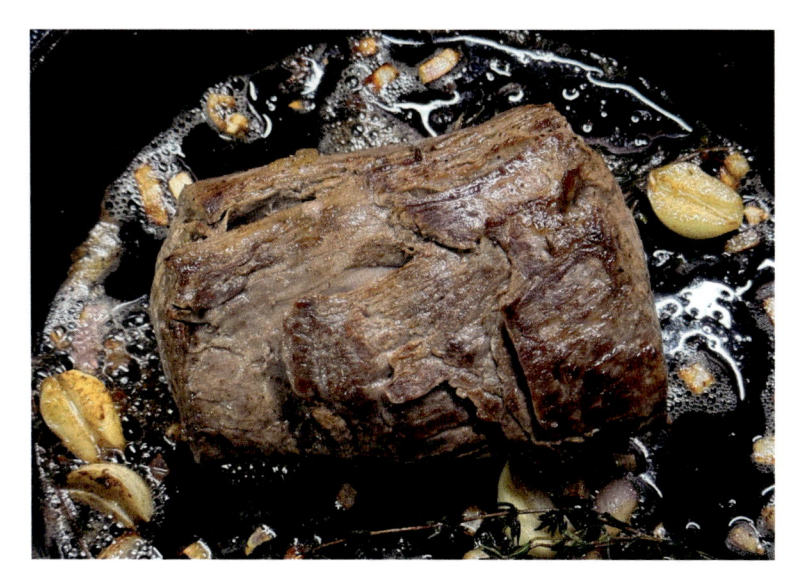

Chateaubriand

An ultra-tender center-cut tenderloin roast from beef, pork, lamb, bison, elk, and even venison

CARB COUNT: 5 GRAMS

INGREDIENTS

2-3 pound fillet mignon roast
1 large shallot, minced
2-5 cloves garlic, smashed
1 stick of butter
3-4 sprigs of thyme
fresh pepper, to taste
16 ounces beef broth
1 tablespoon balsamic vinegar

Notes:
Remove the center sprout from the garlic cloves to avoid bitterness. Traditionally, wine is added to the pan sauce. This is optional.

DIRECTIONS

Dry brine the tenderloin for 2-3 days, then let roast come to room temperature before cooking. Preheat oven to 375°F. Sear roast on all sides in a skillet using animal fat. Add the stick of butter and the herbs to the hot skillet, and baste the roast for a few minutes, as they cook.. Remove meat from skillet and place on a roasting rack, then into the oven for 30-40 minutes until desired temperature is reached (115-120°F for rare, 120-125°F for medium-rare, 130-135°F for medium). The roast will continue cooking as it rests. Allow to rest for 15 minutes before slicing.

While the roast is in the oven, add the broth to the hot skillet, and cook down the liquid to about half. Add in the balsamic. This makes a lovely sauce.

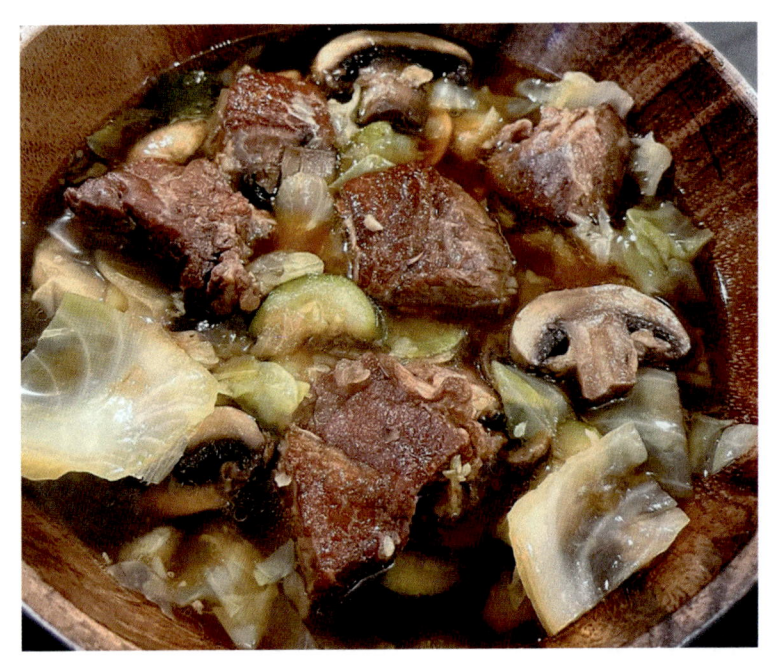

Easy Chuck Roast Soup

CARB COUNT: 18 GRAMS TOTAL

INGREDIENTS

2-3 pounds chuck roast
32 ounces beef broth
1 medium onion, chopped
2 small zucchini, sliced thickly
5 large mushrooms, sliced
½ cabbage (2 cups) chopped
4 garlic cloves, smashed
salt, to taste

DIRECTIONS

After a 2-day dry brine, cube the roast and give the chunks a quick sear in a skillet with animal fat. Place the meat in a pot, Dutch oven, or slow cooker, and add broth or water. In the searing pan, partially cook the onion, adding the garlic near the end to avoid burning it. Add these to the pot and simmer on low, covered, for about 4 hours or until the roast chunks are almost fork tender. Then add the vegetables and continue cooking for another 1-1½ hours, until they are just soft.

Note: The beef can also be shredded with 2 forks.

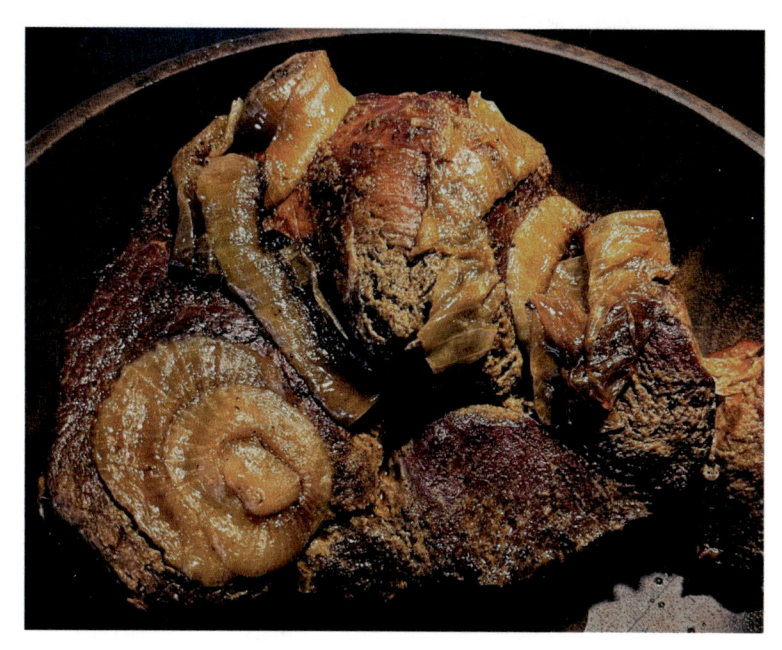

Crockpot Roast

Healthy and nourishing comfort food

CARB COUNT: 0

INGREDIENTS

any roast (see note)
2 cups of broth
salt & pepper
optional:
onions
celery
mushrooms
thyme

DIRECTIONS

Dry brine roast for 1-2 days (see page 3). Sear to brown. Place roast in crock-pot with 2 cups broth and cook covered on low. It takes about 2 hours per pound to reach fork tender, which occurs when the internal temperature reaches over 200°F.

The Instant Pot also works: set to pressure cook on high for 60 minutes for a 3 pound roast (or 10 extra minutes per additional pound). Add an extra 30 minutes if frozen. Natural release for 10 minutes.

Notes: Though chuck and round are ideal, any roast will work: pork, beef, or even a whole chicken. Leftover broth can also be used to make a reduction gravy (page 66) once the roast is done.

Spicy Mongolian Beef

INGREDIENTS

1 pound thinly shaved steak or stir fry beef
½ cup beef stock
¼ cup coconut aminos
1 medium onion
2 tablespoon sesame oil
2 cloves minced garlic
1 tablespoon salt
1 tablespoon black pepper
1 tablespoon crushed red pepper

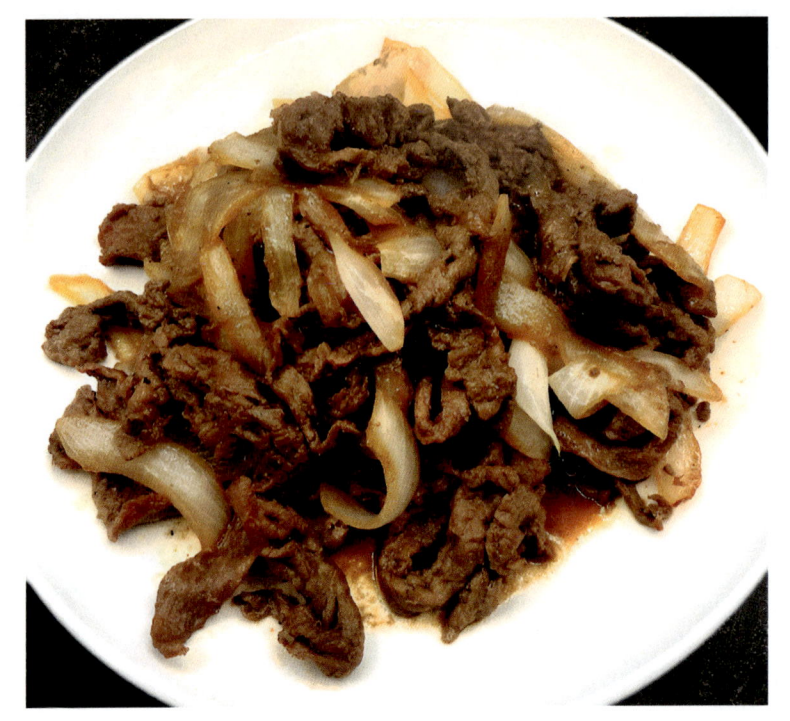

CARB COUNT: 40 GRAMS

DIRECTIONS

Use partially frozen steak and a sharp knife to slice against the grain of the meat in order to achieve thin slices. Marinate the beef overnight or up to 24 hours with all ingredients except the onions. Give a good stir halfway through the marination period. Heat some fat (butter is good) in a skillet, and add the onion chopped into fairly large slices. Cook until they are just turning translucent. Add the beef along with the marinade, and continue cooking until the beef is just done. Avoid overcooking or the beef will tighten up.

Notes: Add cayenne pepper or even more crushed shredded pepper to ratchet up the heat. Though this begs to be served over white rice, or along with broccoli, it's quite satisfying as a stand-alone meal. This recipe makes two very generous sized portions.

Bulgogi Marinade

INGREDIENTS

2 pounds thinly sliced steak
½ cup coconut aminos
¼ cup bone broth
1 tablespoon allulose
2 tablespoons sesame oil
2 tablespoons fresh garlic
1 tablespoon grated ginger (opt.)
1 tablespoon salt
½ teaspoon black pepper
½ teaspoon sesame seeds
red pepper flakes, optional
2 green onions, sliced

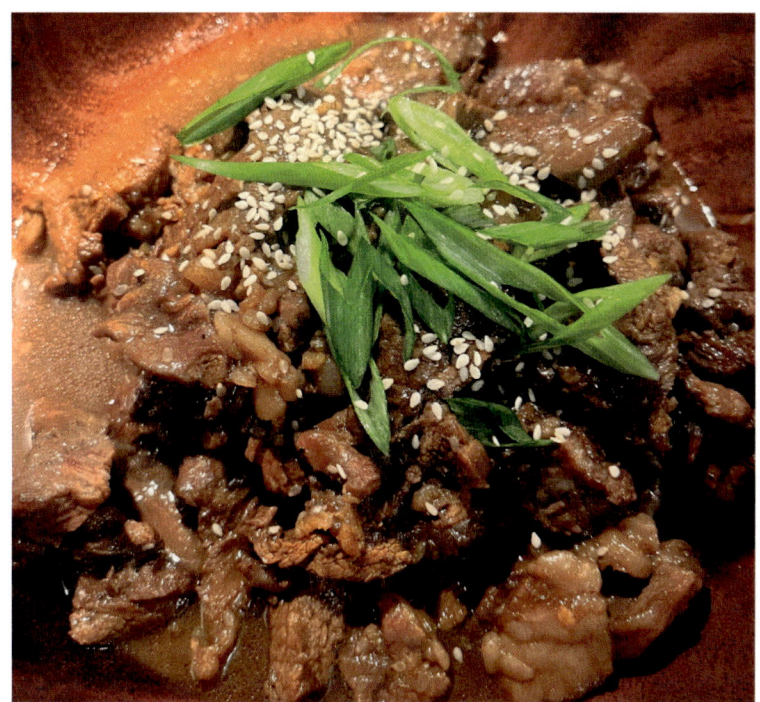

CARB COUNT: 64 GRAMS

DIRECTIONS

Slice semi-frozen beef (preferably ribeye) into thin strips, cutting against the grain. Combine the ingredients, then marinate in glassware for at least 8 hours in the refrigerator. Cook the beef in a skillet on high until done. Garnish with green onions and a sprinkle of sesame seeds.

Notes: Wet meat does not brown, so to get some caramelization, some of the meat can be grilled or pan fried without any marinade. The flavor is better, however, when cooked in the marinade. Adding allulose or sugar to the marinade will help browning. To reduce carbs for this dish, use more broth and less of the coconut aminos (48g carbs)—or limit how much marinade is eaten once prepared. Soy sauce has just as many carbs as coconut aminos. Also, adding 1-2 tablespoons of sweetener gives a more traditional taste.

Oven Ribs

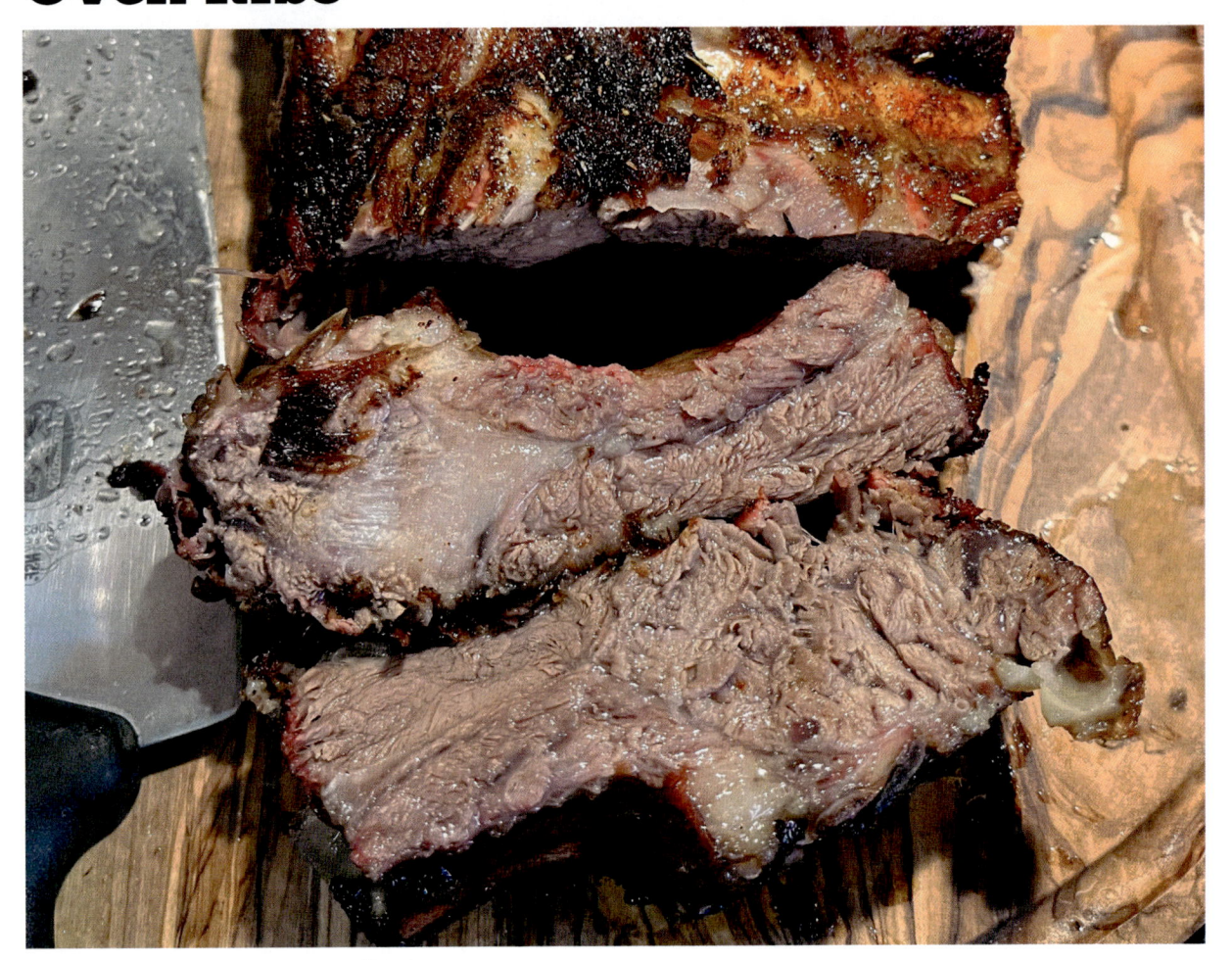

CARB COUNT: 0

Ribs can be made quickly or slowly. What is important is getting the connective tissue to melt so they are tender. Here are two methods that work with either beef or pork, baby back or meaty country style ribs. These can be cooked as slabs, or cut into serving-sized pieces of 2-3 ribs, to fit neatly on a pan.

INGREDIENTS

ribs, beef or pork, any style
favorite rub
BBQ sauce, optional (page 71)

FAST DIRECTIONS

Preheat oven to 400°F. Pat the ribs dry, pull the membrane off the back, and season generously with salt or a rub (easily made with some garlic powder, onion powder, chili powder, paprika, salt, and little cayenne pepper). Place ribs in a baking dish or on a sheet tray and cook uncovered for 45 minutes to an hour.

Notes: The ribs may be seasoned a day in advance, but this isn't necessary. 15 minutes to 24 hours is sufficient.

To fake a smoked flavor, before cooking brush on a mixture of ¼ teaspoon Liquid Smoke, 1 tablespoon Worcestershire sauce, and 1 tablespoon water..

Salt rubs will eat through aluminum foil. Cooking in foil vaporizes aluminum into the food. This should be avoided at all costs.

SLOW DIRECTIONS

Peel the membrane off the back of the ribs and pat dry. Apply a decent dusting of rub mix at least two hours ahead of time. If covering over-night, use parchment paper to cover so meat does not touch foil. Allow ribs to come to room-temperature, about 1 hour.

Set oven to 200°F. Put ribs in meat-side up, covered, using either a stainless pan with sliding lid, another sheet pan upside down as a cover, or parchment followed by foil. Bake for 3-4 hours until internal temperature is 170°F. Turn oven down to 170 or 180°F for 2 more hours to melt the collagen.

Uncover the ribs and drain off juices. They will looked a bit steamed. Baste them in a BBQ sauce and put them under the broiler for 2-3 minutes, then re-coat and re-broil to form a bark. If not using sauce, broil anyway.

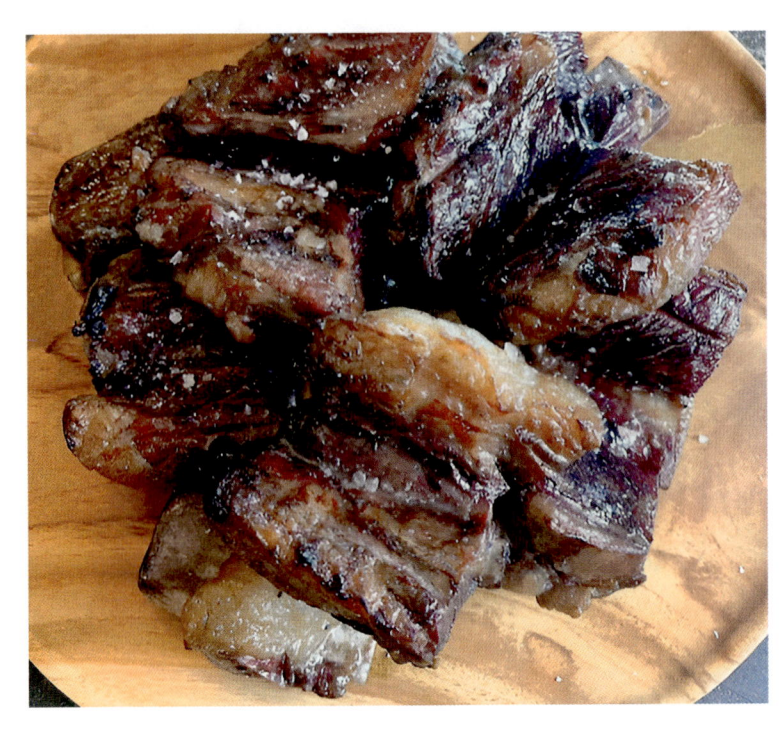

Next-Level Short Ribs

As tender as short ribs can get without braising in liquid

CARB COUNT: 0

INGREDIENTS

beef short ribs
kosher salt

DIRECTIONS

Lightly salt the short ribs all over and dry brine, letting air circulate around them, for 48 hours in the refrigerator. Use a pan with a rack to roast these in the oven at 225°F for 3 hours. The rack is necessary to allow the fat to drip away. Since this is a slow roast, reverse sear the ribs on a grill or in a cast iron pan to brown them up.

Note: Short ribs are ones cut in 2-inch portions. The best ones come from the chuck area. Less expensive and less flavorful short ribs can also come from the brisket, plate, and rib sections.

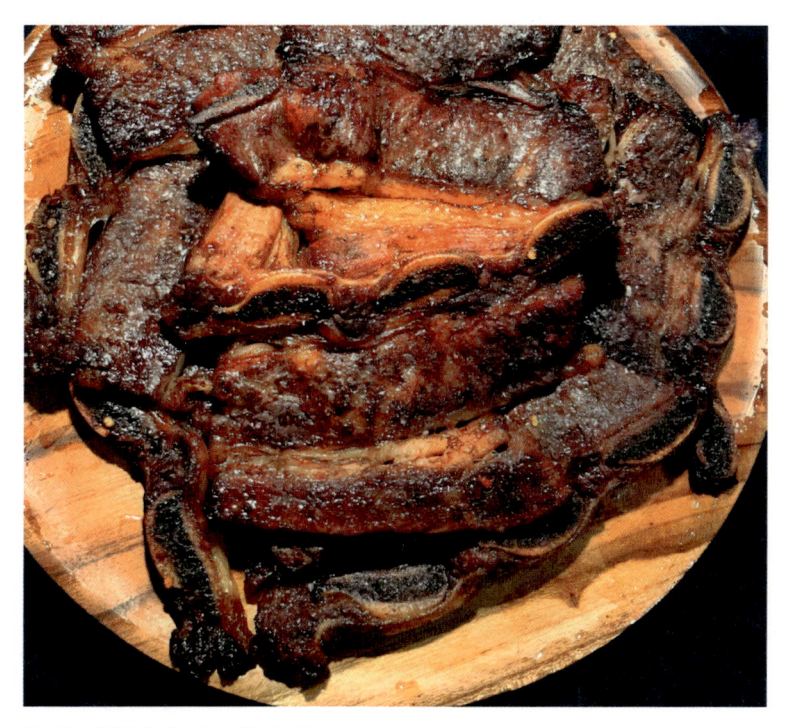

Korean BBQ Short Ribs

Tender and flavorful kalbi

CARB COUNT: 11.4 GRAMS

INGREDIENTS

1 cup coconut aminos
½ cup bone broth
1 tablespoon salt
1 tablespoon sesame oil
½ teaspoon paprika
½ teaspoon garlic powder
½ teaspoon cayenne
½ teaspoon red pepper flakes

DIRECTIONS

Combine all ingredients and marinate flanken style short ribs for 8 to 24 hours. Bake in oven at 375°F for 30 minutes or grill until lightly caramelized.

Note: This marinade makes enough for 2 pounds of ribs. If you don't mind soy, feel free to substitute tamari for the coconut aminos.

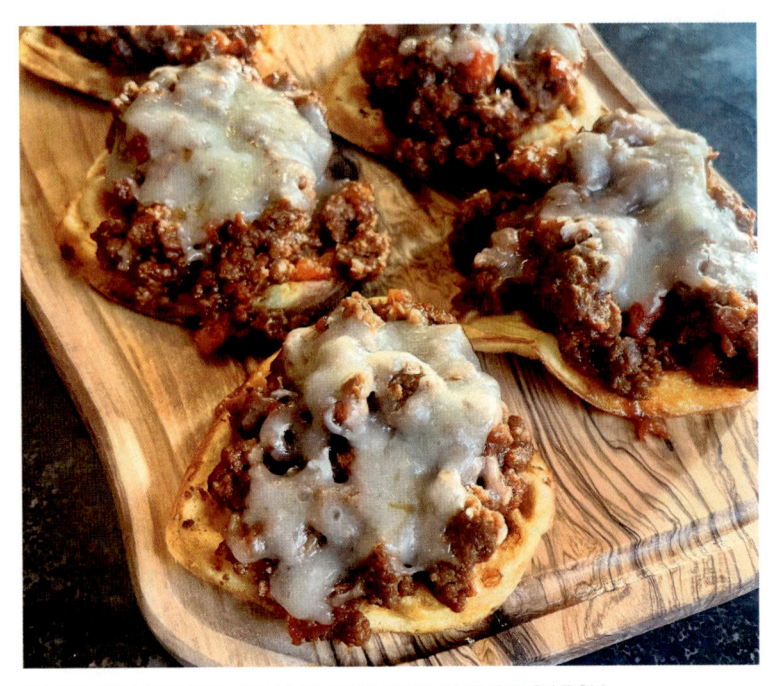

Sloppy Joes

Sometimes you just gotta make some sloppy Joes

CARB COUNT: 19.3 GRAMS FOR THE ENTIRE BATCH

INGREDIENTS

1 pound (500g) ground beef
1 cup (200g) tomato sauce
3 tablespoons tomato paste
3 tablespoons ketchup
1 tablespoon vinegar
1 tablespoon chili powder
½ teaspoon salt
garlic powder
onion powder
provolone cheese

DIRECTIONS

Brown the ground beef then drain the excess fat. Sprinkle the meat with spices, if using. Combine the rest of the ingredients, and simmer briefly. Can be served in a bowl or on a chaffle, topped with shredded or sliced provolone.

Note: These are great in a bowl or on a chaffle bun (page 55) or poured over pork rinds.

Meat-Lovers Chuck Eye Chili

The key to making good chili is to not ruin it with too many veggies.

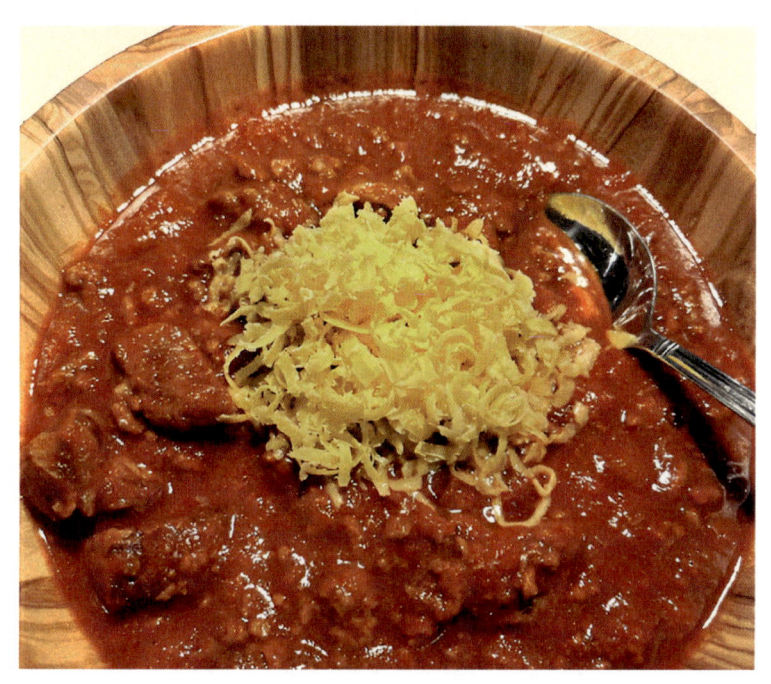

CARB COUNT: 11 GRAMS IN EACH OF 4 SERVINGS

INGREDIENTS

2 pounds cubed or ground meat
1 cup or 1 large onion, chopped
4 cups broth, beef or chicken
14 ounce can diced tomatoes
8 ounce can of tomato sauce
2-4 tablespoons tomato paste
3 tablespoons chili powder
1 tablespoon paprika
1 tablespoon garlic powder
2-3 teaspoons cumin
salt and pepper to taste

DIRECTIONS

Brown the meats in a skillet, drain off excess grease, and add all ingredients to a stock pot. Bring to a boil, then reduce heat and simmer for 1-2 hours, or until desired thickness is reached. Add spices and salt a little at a time to adjust the flavor. Serve topped with cheese or sour cream.

Note: I use a combination of ground chuck and chuck eye steak, and sometimes sausage. Any combination of cubed or ground meat is fine: beef, buffalo, elk, veal, venison, pork, or leftover steak. Even some drained bacon is great. Optional: ½ cup (118 ml) hot sauce or 1 teaspoon cayenne.

Bolognese

This is so good that it stands on its own without pasta.

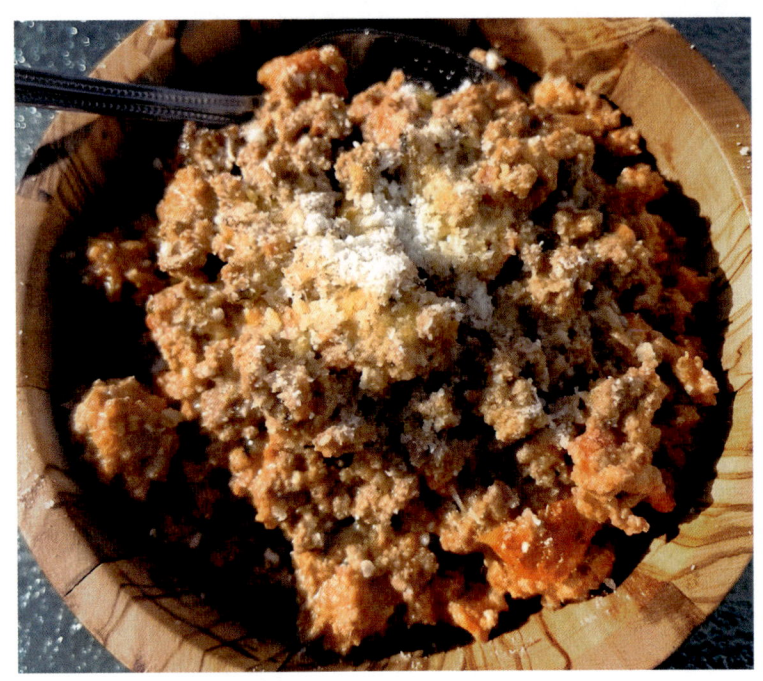

CARB COUNT: 20 GRAMS TOTAL

INGREDIENTS

1 pound (500g) ground beef
½ pound (250g) ground sausage
1 cup (236 ml) heavy cream
2 cups (400g) crushed tomatoes
basil, fresh or dried
oregano, fresh or dried
garlic, fresh or powdered
onion, fresh or powdered
salt to taste
freshly grated hard cheese

DIRECTIONS

Brown the ground beef and sausage, then drain the grease. If using fresh onions and garlic, cook those until soft in a sauté pan with butter or fat. Add all the ingredients, except cheese. Cook on medium heat until desired amount of sauce or thickness is reached, about 20-30 minutes. Finish with grated cheese.

Notes: Bolognese sauce is a classic Italian sauce for pasta. It's thicker than spaghetti sauce, uses dairy, and less tomato. Carrots and celery are a common addition.

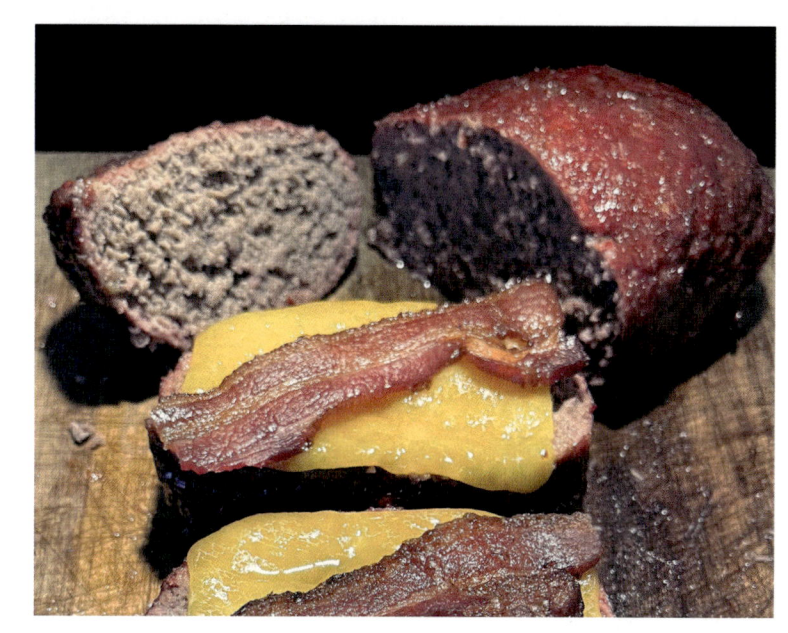

Meatloaf

Mustard and Worcestershire sauce in the mix add nice flavor.

CARB COUNT: ABOUT 13 GRAMS TOTAL

INGREDIENTS

1 (500g) pound ground beef
1 egg
¼ cup (15g) pork rind panko
½ cup (56g) grated Parmesan
2 tablespoons Worcestershire
2 tablespoons yellow mustard
1 tablespoon salt
other seasonings to taste
optional:
garlic and onion powder
red pepper flakes

DIRECTIONS

Combine all ingredients together with hands, then pat to shape. Place loaf on a grated sheet tray or in a special meatloaf pan, if you like the grease to drip out of it. Bake at 350°F for 50-60 minutes.

Meatloaf can be smoked too, for about 2 ½ hours at 180°F. Just turn up the heat to 350°F for the last 20 minutes.

Notes: This can easily become meatballs if you shape them accordingly. This recipe works without the cheese too. Adding 1 teaspoon of gelatin will help retain moisture.

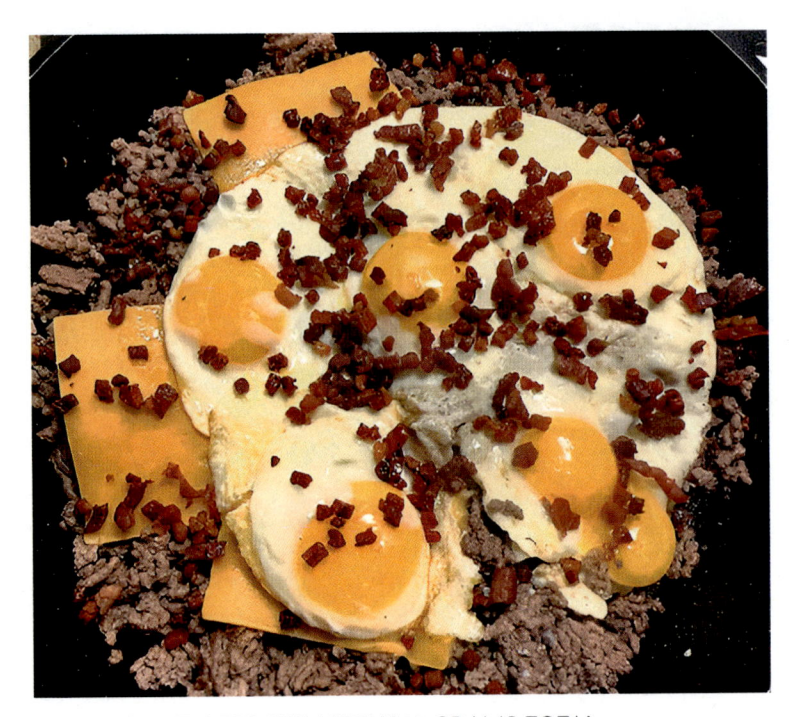

Hamburger Hash

The reliable go to for BBBE: beef, butter, bacon & eggs—plus cheese.

CARB COUNT: APPROXIMATELY 10 GRAMS TOTAL

INGREDIENTS

1 pound ground beef
4 pieces bacon
1 cup (224g) sausage, Italian or Kielbasa
1 cup (113g) cheddar cheese or Tillamook® cheddar slices
over-easy eggs as desired

DIRECTIONS

Brown the ground beef and sausage together, then drain. Cook the bacon and sunny side up eggs separately. Plate the hash first, top with cheddar cheese, then slide the eggs on top. Sprinkle with crumbled bacon or crispy prosciutto.

Notes: A hash is chopped and fried, traditionally made with potato, meat, and onions. This dish is super flexible, and is an inexpensive meal. Adding crispy prosciutto makes it even tastier. The soft egg yolks in this recipe act like sauce and bring it all together.

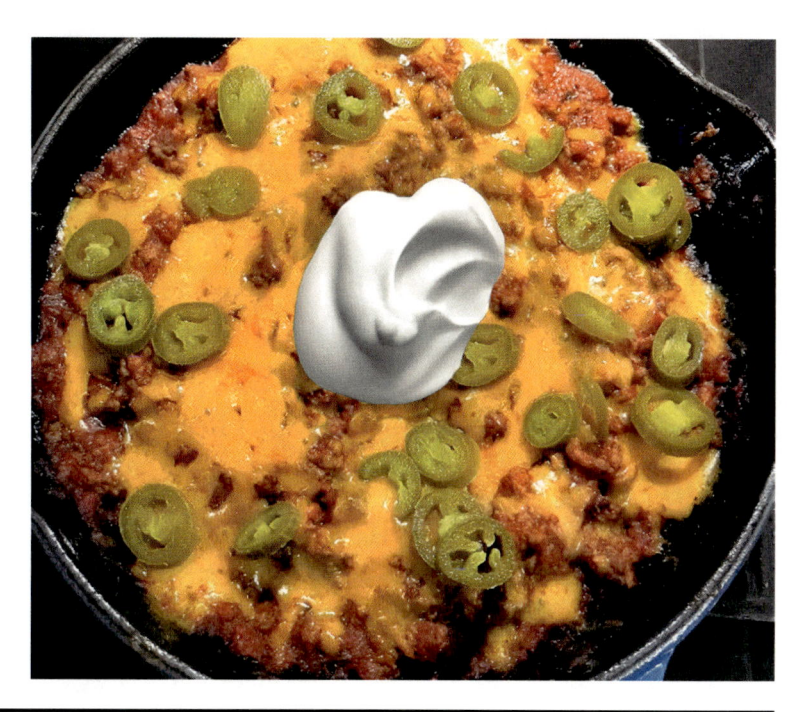

Enchilada Dip

Load up cheese taco shells (page 56) to make enchilacos or taciladas.

CARB COUNT: 17.5 GRAMS TOTAL

INGREDIENTS

1 pound ground beef
2 cups shredded cheddar cheese
12 ounce can tomato sauce
4 ounces goat or cream cheese
½ teaspoon oregano
½ teaspoon paprika
½ teaspoon garlic powder
½ teaspoon onion powder
½ teaspoon salt
½ teaspoon ancho chili powder
¼ teaspoon cayenne pepper
¼ teaspoon cumin

DIRECTIONS

Brown the ground beef and drain the grease. If using fresh onion or garlic, saute them next before adding the tomato sauce and spices to the pan. Use a casserole dish or skillet and spread the goat or cream cheese in the bottom, forming a layer. Top that with the saucy ground beef, and then sprinkle the shredded cheese. Melt in an oven at 350°F, or under the broiler for a few minutes. Garnish with toppings such as jalapeños, green chilies, olives, green or red onions, cilantro, avocado, or sour cream.

Notes: Regular chili powder can be substituted for ancho. Fresh garlic and onions can also be used, Colby Jack too.

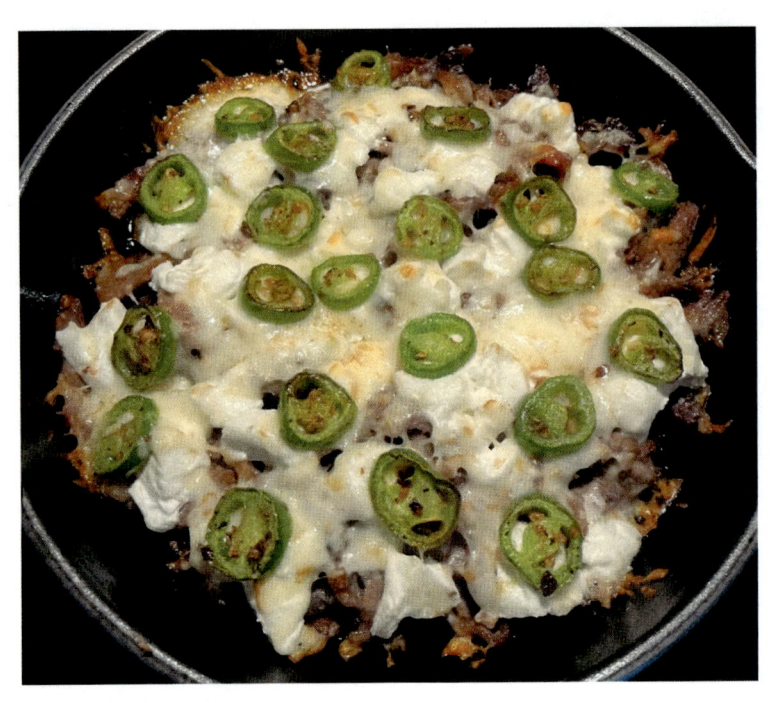

Jalapeño Popper Cheese-Steak

Thinly shaved ribeye puts this over the top.

CARB COUNT: 12 GRAMS

INGREDIENTS

1 pound shaved strip or ribeye
2 cups provolone cheese
4 ounces goat cheese
2 jalapeños

optional:
onions
mushrooms
bell peppers

DIRECTIONS

To get "shaved" meat, take a semi-frozen steak, preferably either strip or ribeye, and slice very thinly with a sharp knife—or have your butcher cut it for you. Set aside meat while slicing and de-seeding the peppers. Cook the peppers (and onions and/or mushrooms) first, lightly in butter or animal fat (bacon grease adds wonderful flavor). Then cook the shaved beef in the skillet. Add the cheeses and jalapeños before melting in a 350°F oven for 10-12 minutes.

Notes: This recipe can be made from start to finish in a small cast iron skillet, though a pie pan also works.

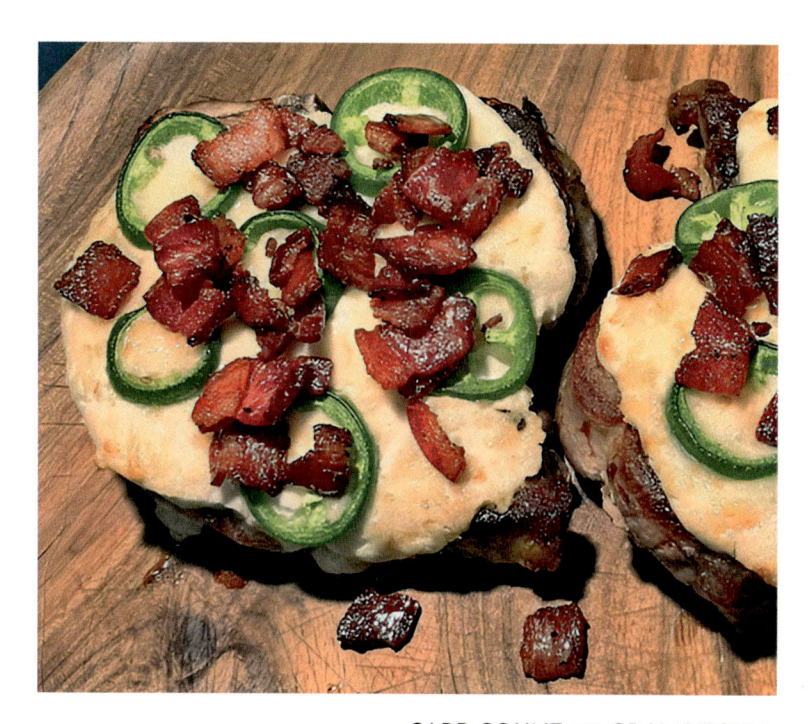

Jalapeño Popper Pork Chop

CARB COUNT: 20 GRAMS TOTAL

INGREDIENTS

3 thick-cut pork chops
8 ounces cream cheese, softened
2 cups shredded cheddar
3 large slices of bacon
3 jalapeños sliced and de-seeded

DIRECTIONS

Preheat oven to 400°F. Pan fry pork chops on medium-high heat in ample fat in a cast iron skillet. While chops are cooking, cut bacon into squares and sauté until crispy in a separate pan. When the internal temperature of the pork chops reach 150°F, spread the tops of the chops with the softened cream cheese. Follow with cheddar and jalapeño slices before transferring the pan to the oven for about 20 minutes. Cook pork until it reaches 165°F to ensure food safety. Serve topped with bacon crumbles.

Smoked Brisket

Keep the fat! Don't trim it off. Let dry brining turn it to magic.

INGREDIENTS

brisket, whole or a smaller cut
kosher salt for dry brining

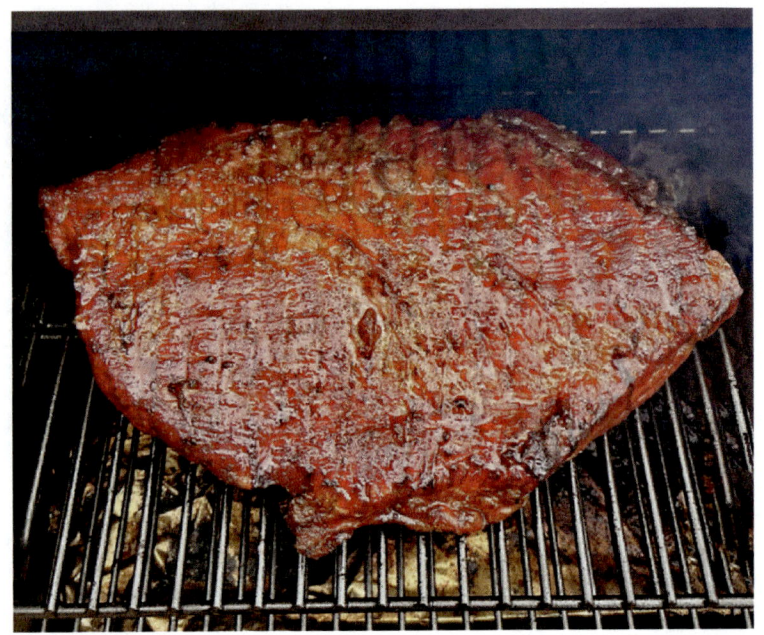

CARB COUNT: 0

DIRECTIONS

Let brisket dry brine for 48 hours in the refrigerator with just plain salt. (See page 3.) Starting with cold meat allows more smoke to cling to the meat surface, so no need to bring it to room temperature first. Put it in a 180°F smoker for about 7 hours, until 152-155°F internally.

Wrap the brisket at this point, first in butcher paper and then foil to enclose it. Keep cooking for an additional 3.5 hours at 250°F until brisket reaches 202°F.

Let it rest in a covered roasting pan or in a cooler for an hour and a half.

Notes: Cooking times will vary with the weight, so go by internal temperatures. A whole brisket weighs between 10 and 16 pounds. From that, the larger cut is the flat, weighing 6 to 10 pounds, while the smaller point cut weighs around 5 to 6 pounds. This brisket was 7.25 pounds.

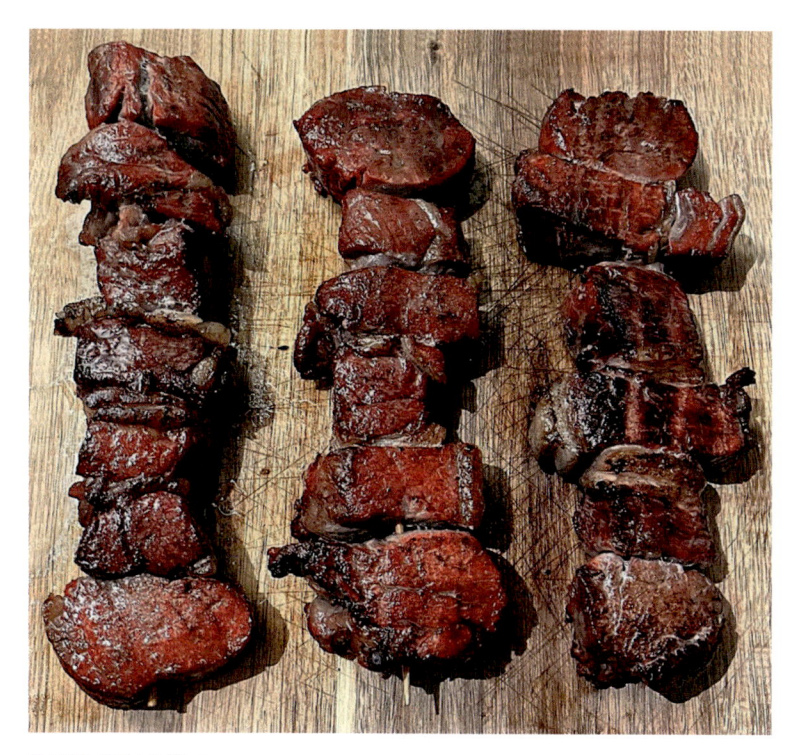

Smoked Kabobs

INGREDIENTS

steak cubed to 2-3"
kosher salt for dry brining

CARB COUNT: 0

DIRECTIONS

Dry brining for 24 hours is really all a good steak needs in terms of a marinade before getting smoked. (See page 3.)

Soak a few wooden skewers before loading them with meat. Get the smoker going at 225°F and smoke the meat for about 1 hour 15 minutes, or until the internal temperature reaches 120°F. Reverse sear in a skillet with ample fat for about 30 seconds on top and bottom. They will sear extremely fast.

Note: Pictured here are filet mignon, ribeye and NY strip.

Smoked Oxtails

These are like meat candy!

INGREDIENTS

2-3 pounds beef or bison oxtails
kosher salt for dry brining

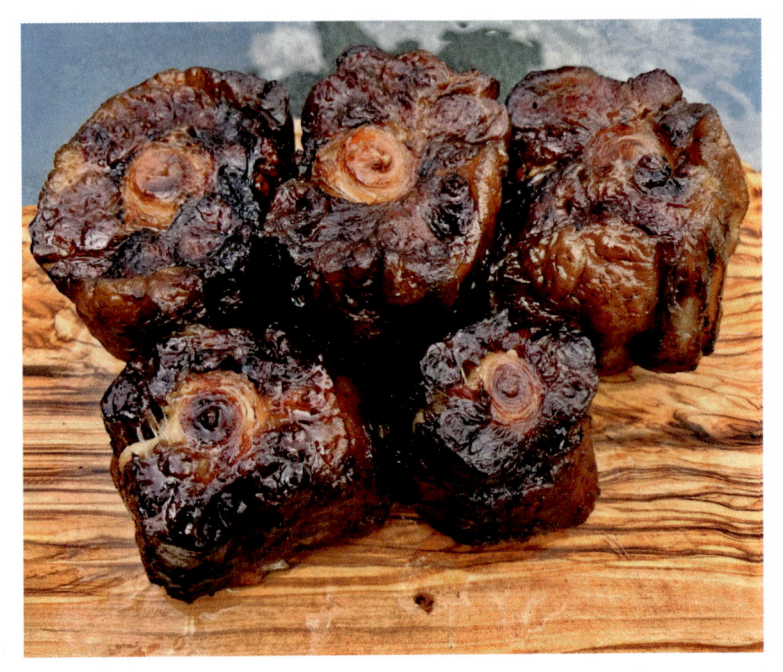

CARB COUNT: 0 GRAMS

DIRECTIONS

Slightly caramelized on the outside, tender on the inside, and barely hanging on the bone! These oxtails begin with a 48-72 hour dry brine.

Smoke at 180°F until their internal temperature reaches 165°F. This takes about four hours. Next place the oxtails in a metal or glass pan. Cover with parchment and then foil, before continuing to cook at 225°F for another 4-5 hours until the internal temperature reaches 202°F.

Notes: There's no reason this method won't work in the oven as well. It also works for ribs and roasts. The key is to aim for the internal temperatures. Cooking times will of course vary.

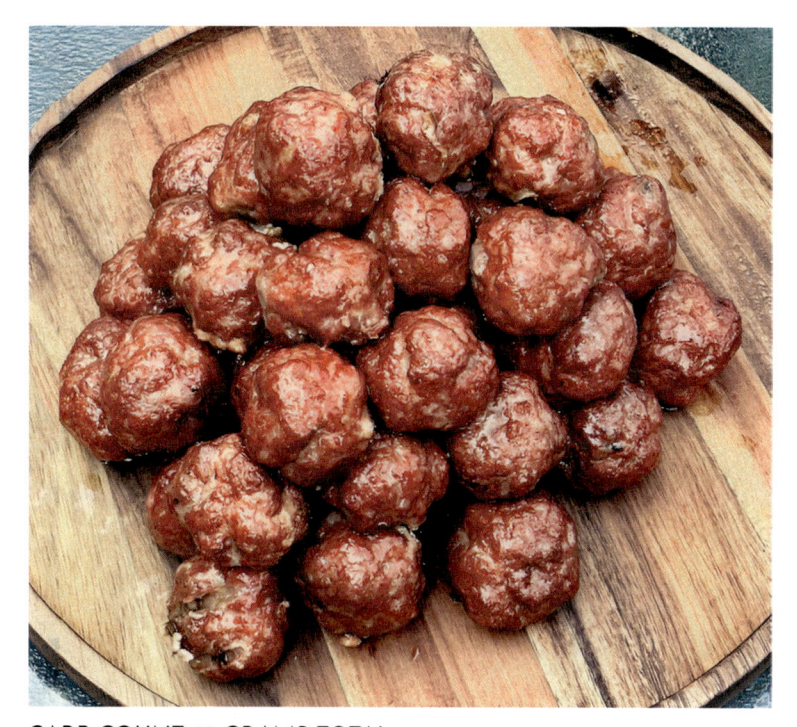

Smoked Meatballs

CARB COUNT: 13 GRAMS TOTAL

INGREDIENTS

1 pound 70/30 ground beef
¼ cup (12g) pork rind crumbs
1 large egg
½ cup grated cheese,
    Parmesan or Romano
2 tablespoons prepared mustard
1 tablespoon Worcestershire sauce
½ teaspoon salt
½ teaspoon garlic powder
½ teaspoon onion powder

DIRECTIONS

Set up your smoker and preheat it to 180°F or 225°F. Whisk the egg, add the seasonings, and combine all ingredients thoroughly in a bowl, but don't ever-work the meat. Use a disher to scoop uniform balls, then using wet hands, smooth into shape. Place the meatballs onto a sheet pan fitted with a rack. Smoke until the internal temperature is around 145-150°F, which should take an hour or two depending on their size and the smoker temperature. Alternatively, they can be baked at 350°F in an oven for about 30 minutes. (For faking smoke flavor, see page 14 in the rib section.)

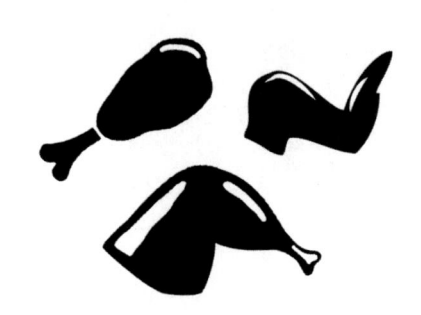

Poultry Dishes

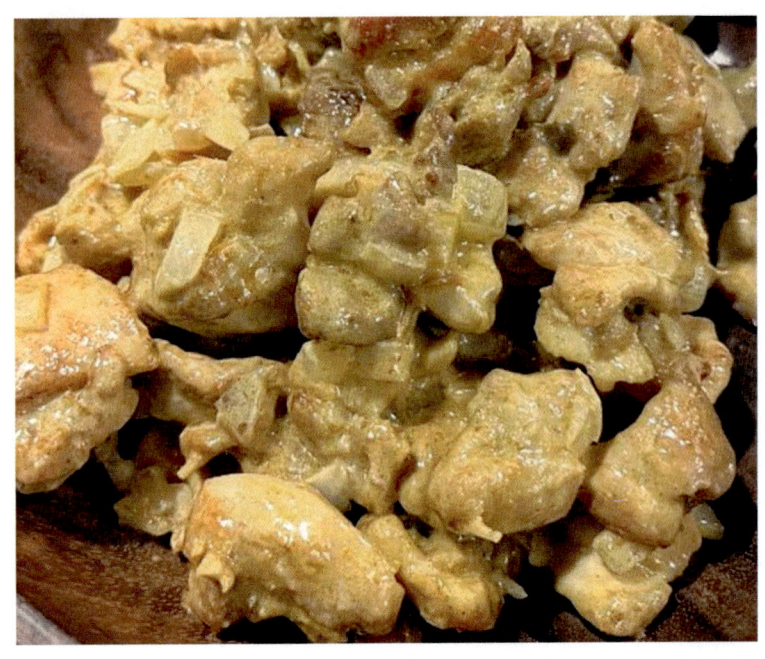

Butter Chicken

A very easy and flexible curry!

CARB COUNT: 11 GRAMS

INGREDIENTS

1 pound boneless chicken thighs
2 teaspoons salt
1 ½ teaspoons turmeric
1 teaspoon ground ginger
1 teaspoon chili powder
1 teaspoon garam masala
½ teaspoon paprika
½ teaspoon cayenne (optional)

½ cup heavy cream
½ medium onion
3 tablespoons butter

DIRECTIONS

Cut the chicken into large bite-sized pieces. Sprinkle with seasonings, mixing thoroughly. Cover and let refrigerate overnight in glassware. Cook chicken in a skillet with a little animal fat. Add the diced onion and one tablespoon of butter. If using garlic, add it after the onions. When chicken is fully cooked, and onion is soft, add 2 tablespoons of butter along with the cream. Keep stirring on medium heat until sauce comes together. This should take 1-2 minutes.

Note: Too much butter can break the sauce emulsion, and so can reheating. This might be avoided if cream is added when reheating in a skillet.

Buffalo Chicken Dip

This is a great dip for pork rinds, and a good use for leftover chicken—especially the boring breast meat.

INGREDIENTS

2 cups shredded cooked chicken (4 medium thighs or 2 breasts)
1 cup heavy cream
4 ounces blue cheese
8 ounces goat cheese
¼-½ cup hot sauce, Frank's
salt to taste

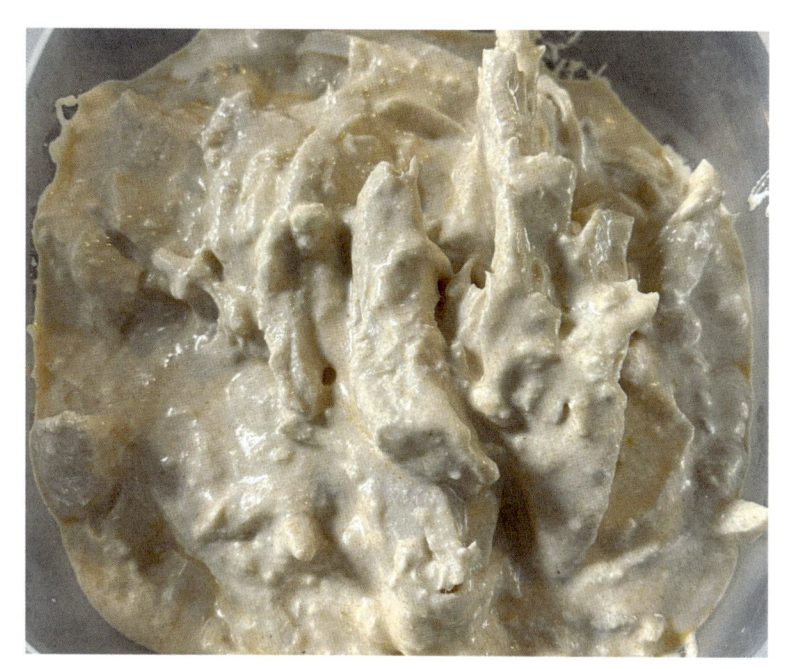

CARB COUNT: 13 GRAMS

DIRECTIONS

If you don't have leftover chicken, prepare some boneless skinless thighs or breasts to make the dip. This can be done by **baking** at 350°F for 35-40 minutes until 165°F internally, or in an Instant Pot. Shred the chicken by pulling at it with two forks to separate the fibers.

Instant Pot variation: Add 2 tablespoons of butter if using breasts. It's not necessary to sear the chicken first, just put it in the pot with 1 cup of liquid, like broth and some hot sauce. Season chicken with salt and garlic powder, add paprika for more color and flavor. Pressure cook on high for 10-15 minutes, and use either manual or natural release. You can also simmer the broth down to concentrate it, especially if you added hot sauce. Chicken can be shredded in the juices.

To make the dip: Use a saucepan to heat 1 cup of cream on medium-low and add the cheeses. Stir gently until melted, then add the shredded chicken and hot sauce—to taste.

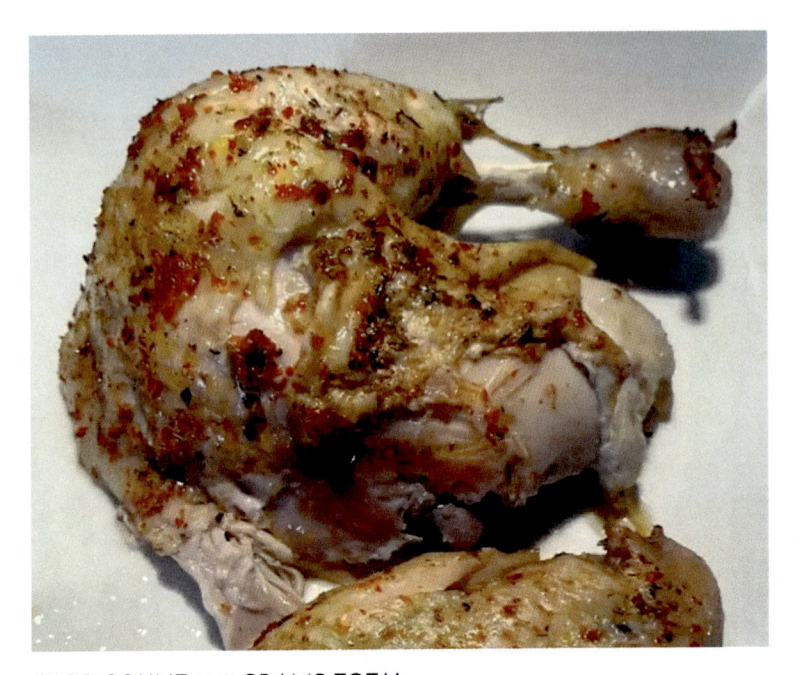

Spicy Korean Chicken

CARB COUNT: 6-8 GRAMS TOTAL

INGREDIENTS

1 whole chicken
1 cup of chicken stock
¼-½ cup course bidan red pepper or other red pepper flakes
1 teaspoon garlic powder
1 teaspoon onion powder
1-2 teaspoons salt

DIRECTIONS

Sprinkle bird generously with salt, garlic, onion, and red pepper flakes (to taste). Place into Instant Pot along with one cup of broth. Secure lid and set pressure cooking time for about 30 minutes. Use a natural pressure release. To crisp up the skin, the bird can be placed on a tray and roasted in a 450°F oven for about 10 minutes. Be sure to save the broth, it's delicious. The flavor is complex with a slow heat.

Note: Bidan (gochugaru) Korean spicy red pepper is available through Amazon. It's the kind traditionally used to make Kim Chi. It's slightly sweet and smoky in addition to its spiciness.

Fried Chicken

100% carnivore too!

INGREDIENTS

chicken pieces, any
gelatin powder
beaten egg
pork panko, seasoned or plain
optional: salt, pepper, garlic, onion
tallow or lard for frying

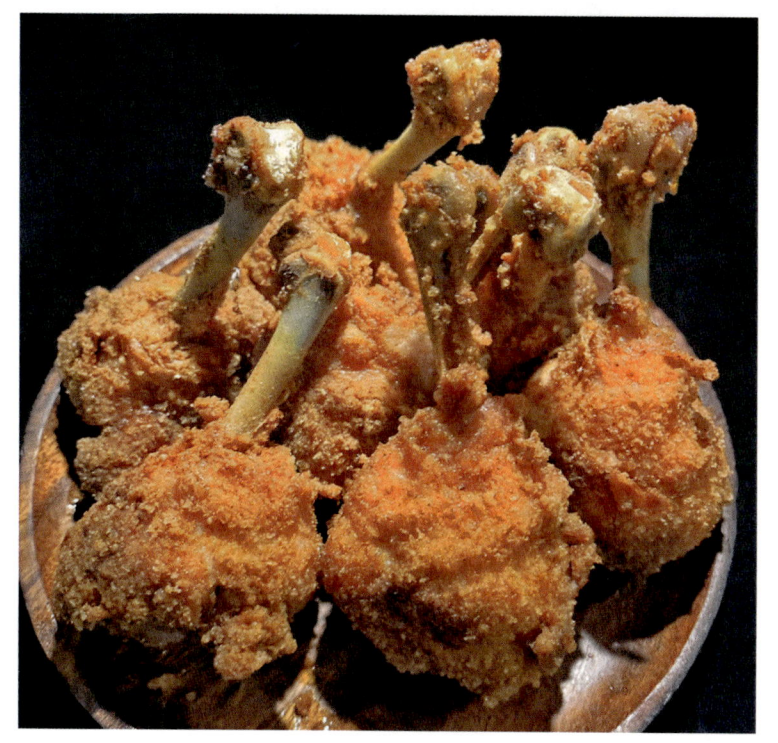

CARB COUNT: 1 GRAM TOTAL

DIRECTIONS

This works with boneless skinless, pounded chicken, or bone-in with skin parts. You can start by dry-brining your favorite chicken cut (bone-in and skin-on is best) in one teaspoon of salt per pound of chicken, overnight in the refrigerator, but this is optional.
Pat the chicken dry, sprinkle lightly with gelatin powder, then dip into a bowl of beaten eggs. Shake off any excess before dipping into a bowl with pork panko crumbs. Proceed to fry in a hot skillet using animal fat. Keep the heat low when frying—no hotter than 325°F. Try not to crowd the pieces in the pan, and be careful when turning them so as not to bruise the breading.

Note: Pictured is lollipop cut chicken which is a Frenched chicken drummette from the wing.

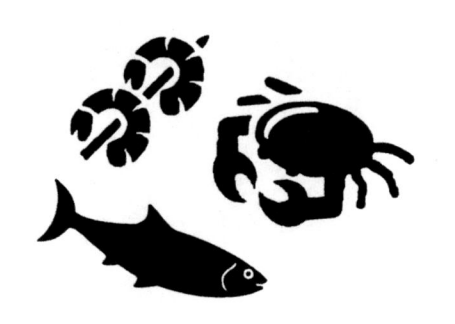

Seafood

Maryland Style Shrimp

McCormick's Old Bay Seasoning is the key. This hits the spot for a spicy food craving. Serve hot or cold.

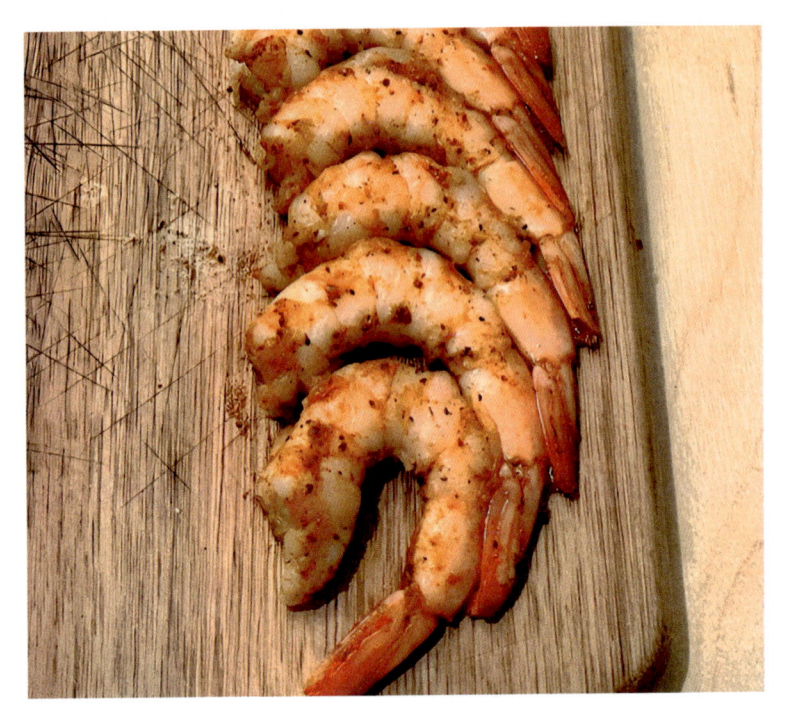

CARB COUNT: 8.5 GRAMS PER POUND

INGREDIENTS

1-2 pounds of shrimp
2-4 tablespoons Old Bay
optional, cayenne pepper

Notes: If you don't have Old Bay, Cajun seasoning is an alternative. Other recipes use cider vinegar and beer in the cooking water.

DIRECTIONS

Select shrimp, jumbo or extra-large work best for tossing with seasonings. Fresh are ideal, but frozen are convenient. Choose either pre-cooked, or raw deveined, which will save a few dollars. You can cook these from frozen. Bring a pot of water to a boil and toss the shrimp in for 3-4 minutes. Cool them down immediately in a cold or ice water bath. Peel the shrimp, and then toss with spices. Use 2 tablespoons of Old Bay seasoning for every pound of shrimp. If you prefer them spicier, add some cayenne.

Crab Stuffed Shrimp

Use the crab cake recipe on page 40 to stuff a few shrimp.

CARB COUNT: 12.5 GRAMS TOTAL or 0.5 GRAMS EACH

INGREDIENTS

1 ½ pounds of 16-20 count shrimp, raw, de-veined, any color
8 ounces lump white crab meat
1 large egg, beaten
¼ cup pork panko crumbs
4 ½ teaspoons grated Parmesan
1-2 teaspoons Old Bay Seasoning

Note: There's no need to spring for the expensive jumbo lump crab or go cheap with claw meat.

DIRECTIONS

Thaw and peel the shrimp, leaving the shell on the delicate tail. De-vein if necessary and slice a little deeper along there so the shrimp can be butterflied (spread out) to hold some filling. Preheat oven to 375°F. With the crab meat in a bowl, sprinkle with seasoning, Parmesan, and pork panko, then mix it up a bit before combining with the beaten egg. Use a tablespoon to gently saddle a dollop of crab mix onto the waiting shrimp. Arrange on a baking sheet lined with parchment paper, and bake for 20-25 minutes until golden and crispy.

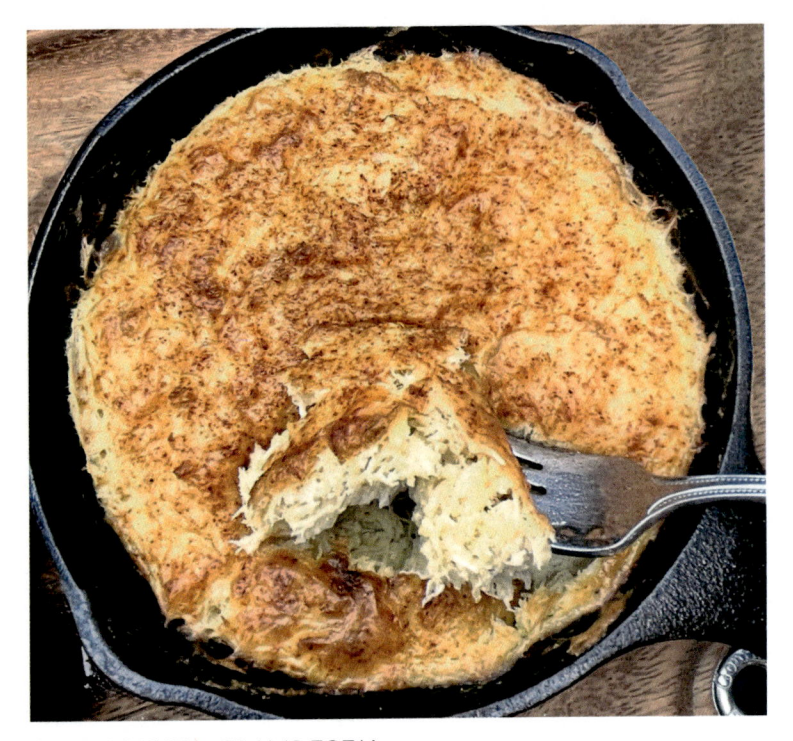

Smoked Crab Imperial

You can choose to not bake this too and it will be a delicious crab salad.

CARB COUNT: 2 GRAMS TOTAL

INGREDIENTS

2 cups crab meat
4 tablespoons melted butter
3 egg yolks
2 ounces goat cheese
to taste:
salt
Old Bay Seasoning
garlic powder
onion powder

DIRECTIONS

First make butter mayo with goat cheese by melting the butter, adding room temperature egg yolks and goat cheese then combining with an immersion blender in a bowl. This is delicious all by itself!

Combine this with the crab meat and seasonings. Then scrape this into a small baking dish. If you have a smoker, preheat it and try 350°F for about 20 minutes with a wood like apple. If you only have an oven, then go ahead and bake 350°F for about 20 minutes.

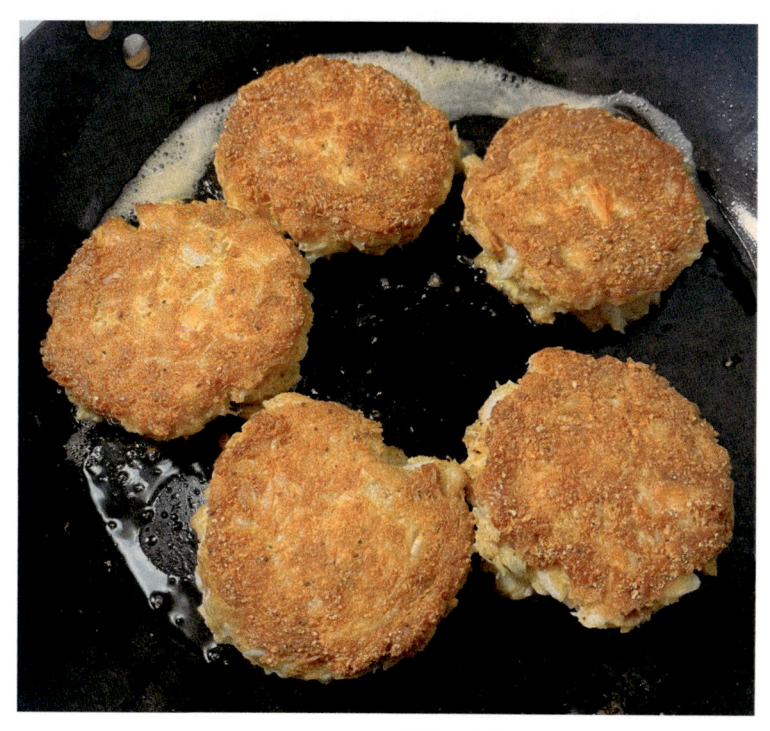

Crab Cakes

Simple is better when it comes to keto crab cakes.

CARB COUNT: 6 GRAMS TOTAL

INGREDIENTS

1 pound can of lump crab meat
2 raw eggs, scrambled
½ cup pork panko crumbs
3 tablespoons grated Parmesan
3-4 teaspoons Old Bay

DIRECTIONS

Whisk two eggs in a mixing bowl, then add all ingredients and mix well. Form into 8-10 patties. Pan fry the cakes over medium heat in a skillet with plenty of animal fat, 3 minutes per side.

Note: A simple garlic butter goes well as a dipping sauce. This mix can be used to stuff shrimp too.

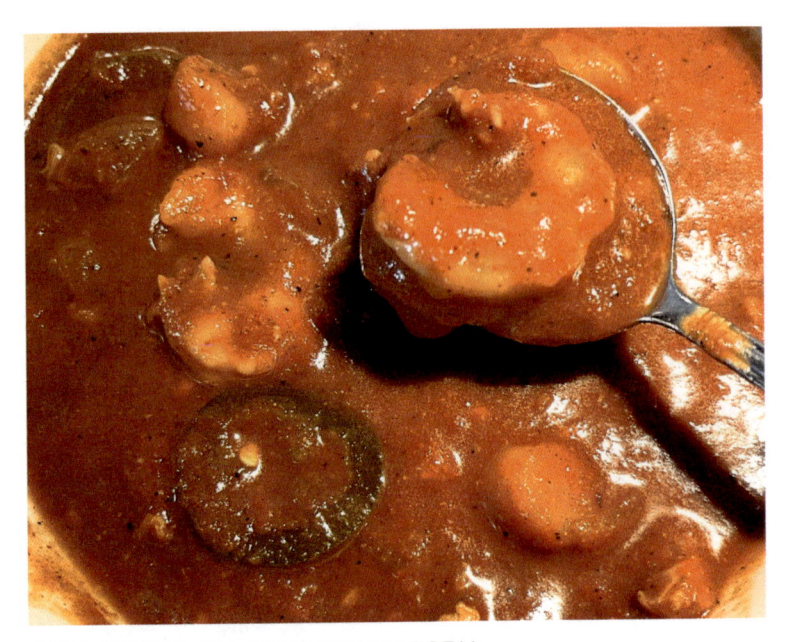

Seafood Chili

Clam juice really brings out the seafood flavor so it's not lost in the chili.

CARB COUNT: ABOUT 70 GRAMS TOTAL

INGREDIENTS

2 pounds of mixed seafood: clams, scallops, shrimp
6 cups clam juice
12 ounces tomato sauce
2 cups diced tomatoes
2-4 tablespoons tomato paste
1 jalapeño, seeded and chopped
1 small onion, chopped
2 tablespoons chili powder
1 teaspoon paprika
1 teaspoon garlic powder*
½-1 teaspoon cumin
salt and pepper

DIRECTIONS

In a pot, sauté the onions and jalapeño in a bit of fat. Add the tomato ingredients along with the spices. Let this cook down, allowing the flavors to meld for about 10 minutes. Next add the seafood items and the clam juice. Bring to a quick boil, then reduce heat and simmer for 5-10 minutes. You do not want to overcook the delicate seafood.

Note: This is good with 4 fresh cloves of garlic, and served with a bit of lime juice squeezed on top.

*If not using fresh garlic, add the garlic powder to the clam juice rather than directly into the tomatoes.

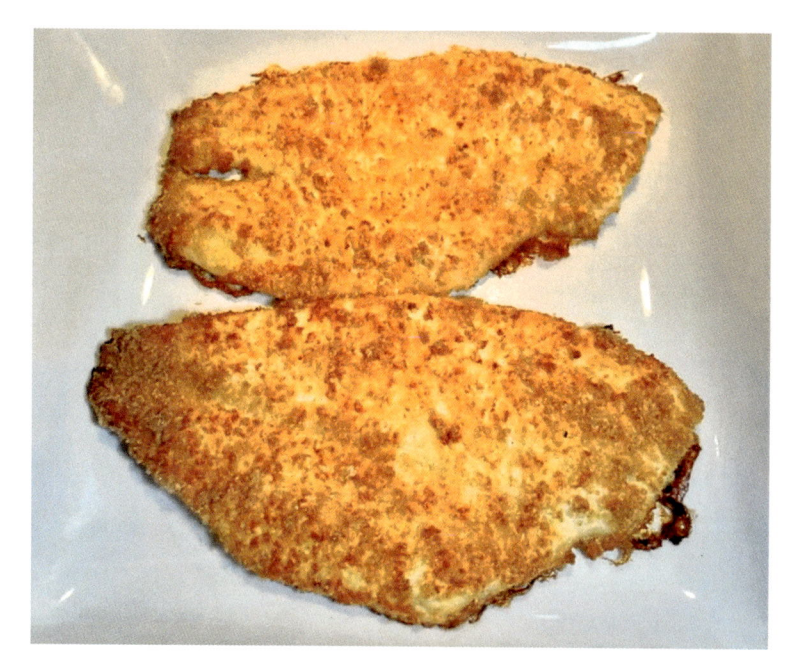

Breaded Flounder

This method works great for other fish as well.

CARB COUNT: 0.5 GRAMS

INGREDIENTS

fresh flounder fillets
gelatin powder
1 raw egg, whisked in a bowl
pork panko crumbs
garlic powder
salt

DIRECTIONS

Dry fresh fish on unbleached paper towels for 15 minutes before breading. If you need to make some pork panko, add pork rinds to a food processor and pulverize briefly. I like 4505 brand. Take the gelatin powder and sprinkle it lightly over the fish. A cheese shaker jar works well for this. Next, take hold of the fish and dip it into the egg with one hand. Shake excess egg off before dredging the fish into the pork panko bowl, being sure to get good coverage. Lay the fishes onto a parchment lined baking sheet, and season to taste with garlic and salt. Bake at 425°F for 20-25 minutes, depending on the size of your fish. (For cod, use 400°F for 40 minutes.)

Eggs

No-Mayo Deviled Eggs

All the goodness with none of the guilt of seed oils

CARB COUNT: 0.9 GRAMS EACH

INGREDIENTS

6 boiled eggs
4 tablespoons bone broth
1 ½ tablespoons butter
1 tablespoon white vinegar
salt, to taste
optional:
½-1 tablespoons yellow mustard
garlic & onion powder
paprika
bacon or pork belly bits

DIRECTIONS

Boil the eggs for 10-12 minutes, then cool under running water. Once cooled, carefully peel and then cut the eggs in half the long way. Scoop the yolks into a bowl as well as the white portion from two of the eggs. Add the butter, broth, vinegar, water, mustard (if using), and any seasonings. Mix with an immersion blender or food processor until smooth. Spoon, scoop, or pipe the mixture to fill the white halves, into little mounds. Top dress with chopped bacon or pork belly bits. Dust with paprika for added color.

Note: Using mustard will make the eggs tangier. Chives cut into tiny rings add flavor and contrast. Recipe makes 4.

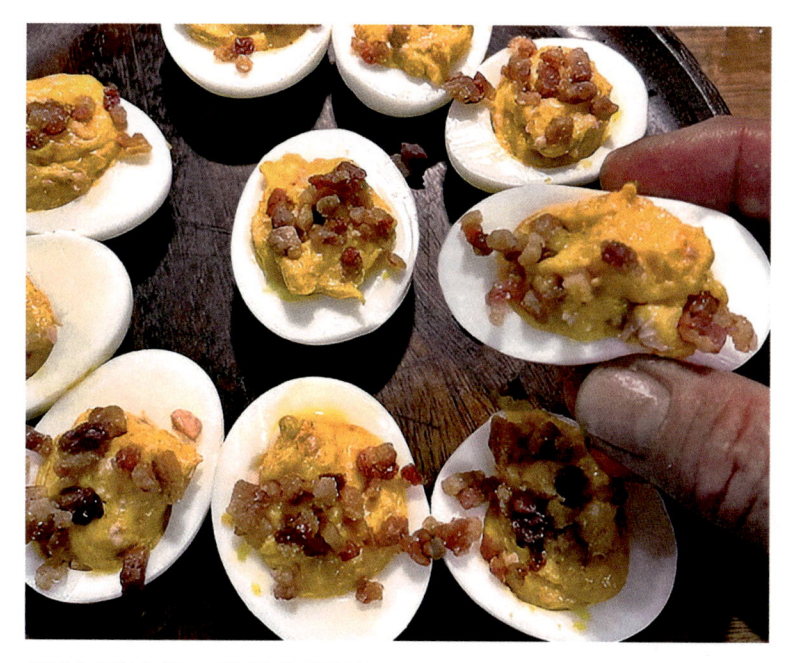

Cod Liver Deviled Eggs

A delicious way to hide liver in eggs.

CARB COUNT: 3 GRAMS TOTAL

INGREDIENTS

4 ounce can (113g) cod livers in oil
5 medium to hard boiled eggs
bacon or pork belly bits
salt to taste

Note: To reduced the taste of the cod liver (which is quite similar to anchovies), add more egg yolks.

DIRECTIONS

Boil the eggs for 10-12 minutes, then cool under running water. Once cooled, carefully peel and then cut in half long ways. Scoop the yolks into a bowl. Combine the cod livers with the cooked yolks, add about half of the oil from the tin. Mix with a fork to the desired consistency, adding more oil if necessary. Spoon or pipe the mixture to fill the white halves, creating little mounds. Top dress with bacon or pork belly bits. Chives cut into tiny rings look attractive as well as add flavor.

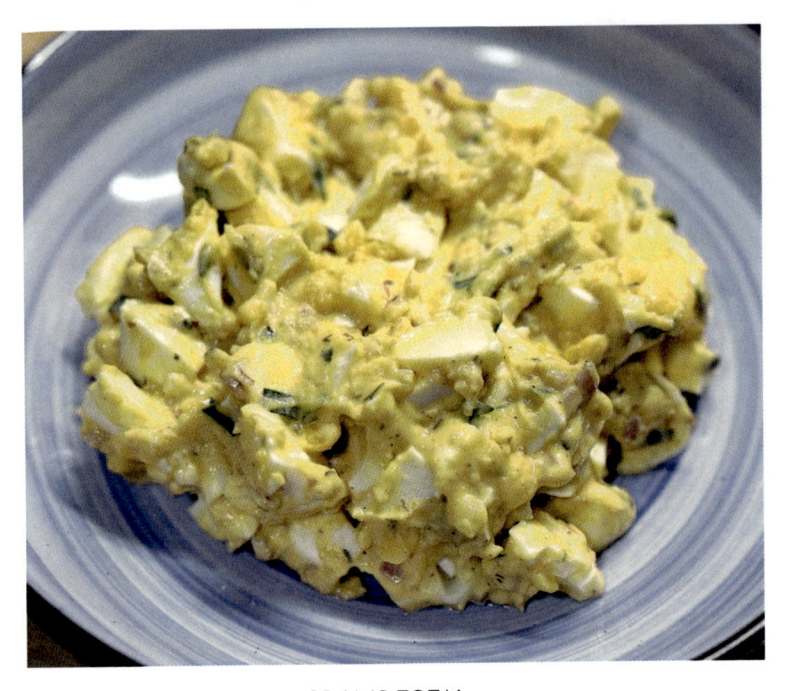

Egg Salad

A good way to use up hard boiled eggs and extra mayo

CARB COUNT: ABOUT 6 GRAMS TOTAL

INGREDIENTS

6 large eggs, hard boiled
1 small shallot minced
¼ cup mayo or aioli
1 tablespoon Dijon mustard
1-2 teaspoons hot sauce
¼ teaspoon salt
fresh pepper

DIRECTIONS

Eggs can be boiled days in advance. Use firmly set eggs, but not overcooked either. Peel, them then roughly chop and set aside. Dice the eggs as finely or coarsely as you like. Mix the saucy ingredients together in a bowl before stirring in the chopped eggs. This can be eaten right away, but is even better after an hour or two. It will keep for about 5 days in the refrigerator.

Notes: Soft yolks can lead to runny dressing. Some people like to add celery bits for crunchy texture, but the shallot offers that too with better flavor. Use the version of mayonnaise you prefer.

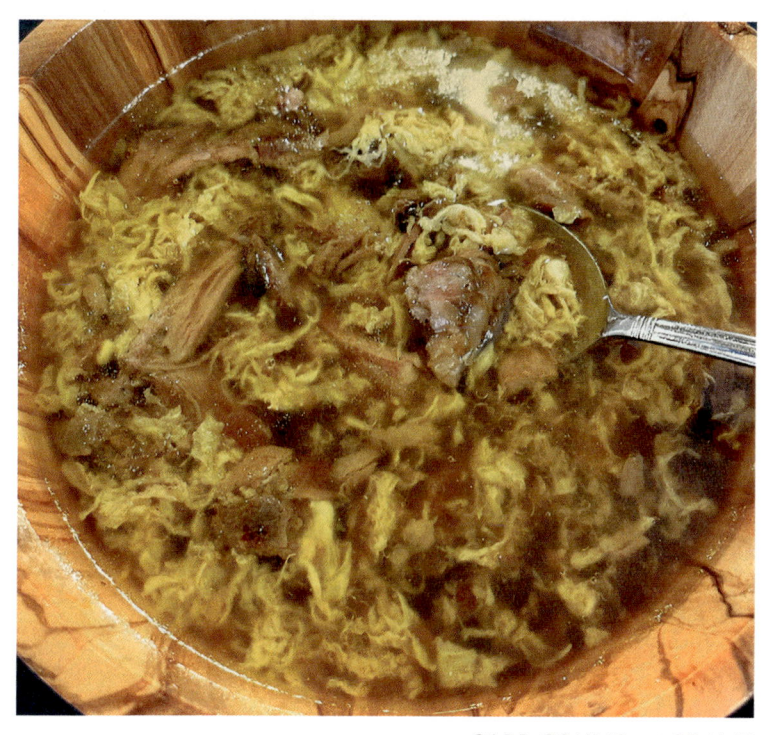

Egg Drop Soup

CARB COUNT: 1.5 GRAMS

INGREDIENTS

2 cups (473 ml) chicken broth
1 scrambled egg
optional:
garlic powder
black or white pepper
shredded meat
green onions

DIRECTIONS

Bring broth to a boil in a small sauce pan then reduce heat to a simmer. Make a whirlpool in the broth by stirring with a whisk or spoon, and slowly pour the beaten egg in a thin stream. The egg will cook upon contact with hot broth, forming fine ribbons while being stirred. Season with garlic and onion powder or even thyme. Garnishing with fresh chives is also nice.

Notes: Restaurants use turmeric for enhanced color, corn starch for thickening, and sesame oil for flavoring, which is unnecessary. This is a perfect light meal, pictured here with leftover roast.

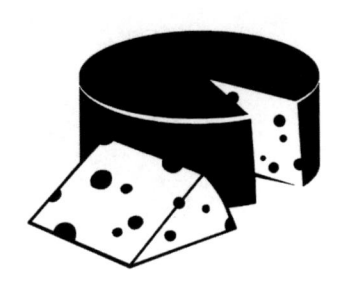

Cheese Magic

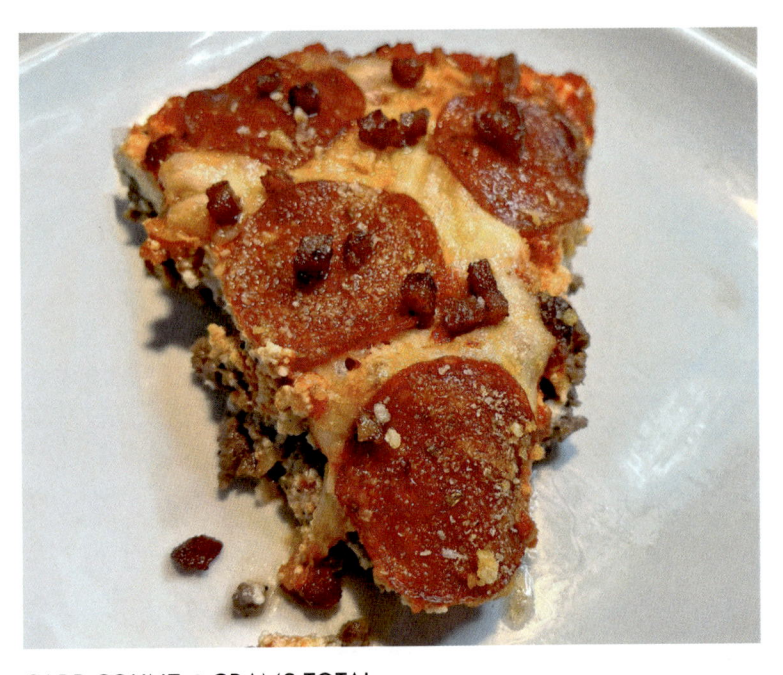

Pizzagna

Layered deep dish lasagna pizza

CARB COUNT: 8 GRAMS TOTAL

INGREDIENTS

1 pound ground beef
½ pound ground sausage
2 cups (500g) ricotta cheese
1 ¼ cups crushed tomatoes
2 eggs
2 cups (226g) mozzarella
pepperoni slices
Italian spices, to taste

DIRECTIONS

Preheat oven to 350°
Pre-cook the meats and drain off grease. Place meat in the bottom of a casserole dish, 10" cake pan, or cast iron skillet. Combine the ricotta with the eggs, then spread that on top of the meats. Drain the crushed tomatoes well before adding them. Sprinkle the cheese, then top with pepperoni. Bake for 30-35 minutes. Let the dish cool for 15 minutes to firm up before serving.

Notes: Italian seasonings and spicy sausage are nice additions. Pizza sauce usually has basil, garlic, and oregano in it, which can be added with the meat. Extra ricotta and shredded cheese do not hurt this dish. Add other toppings as desired.

Cheesehead Pizza

A fat bomb that hits like cheesy bread, but satisfies like pizza

CARB COUNT: 22 GRAMS TOTAL

INGREDIENTS

2 ½ cups (282g) mozzarella
2 eggs
½ cup (56g) grated Parmesan
1 tablespoon melted butter
½ cup (73g) pepperoni slices

DIRECTIONS

Combine 2 eggs with the ½ cup of grated Parmesan and 2 cups shredded cheese (any kind really, but be sure to save half a cup of shredded mozzarella for topping after the crust is cooked). Place on a parchment lined sheet tray, and bake at 350°F for 15-20 minutes. Add melted butter as sauce, the remaining cheese and the pepperoni. Bake for an additional 8-10 minutes.

Notes: You can add no-sugar crushed tomatoes as a sauce and any additional toppings like sausage, diced ham, olives, or mushrooms. Garlic and Italian seasonings may also be included.

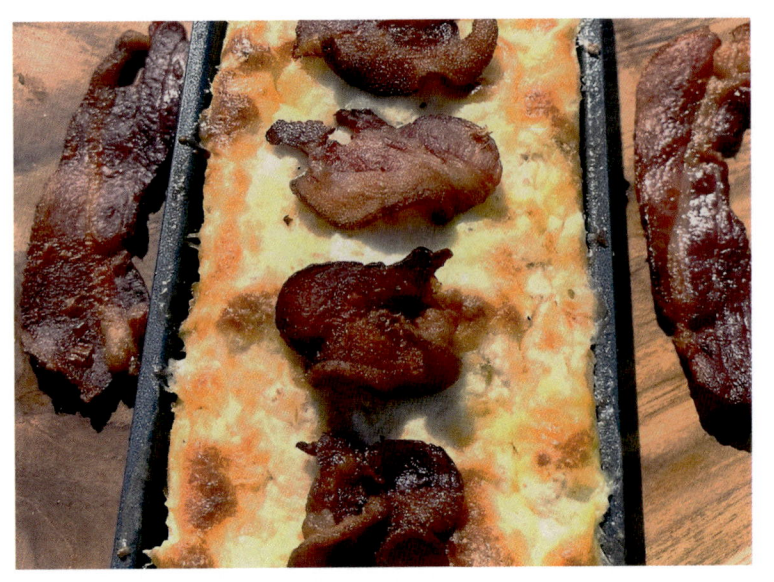

Breakfast Lasagna

Yes, lasagna is a casserole, but this one does not have pasta.

CARB COUNT: 10-15 GRAMS TOTAL

INGREDIENTS

½-¾ lb ground sausage
4-6 eggs, beaten
4-6 oz (113-170g) ricotta cheese
½-¾ cup shredded cheese
4+ bacon slices (or more)
salt and pepper
red pepper flakes (optional)
garlic powder (optional)
fresh thyme (optional)

DIRECTIONS

First cook sausage and bacon separately, then drain while pre-heating oven to 350°F. Grease a loaf pan with butter, and spread a layer of sausage on the bottom. Pour the beaten eggs over the cooked sausage. If adding spices, mix them in with the eggs. Make a layer of ricotta. Bacon can be added as a layer, or used only as a decoration. Top with shredded cheese. Bake for 25-30 minutes, and garnish with bacon before serving.

Notes: Loaf pans vary, so scale the recipe up or down as needed. Using more shredded cheese will create a nice cap on the loaf. Bacon pieces in the loaf will be chewy and tender, similar to noodles. They can be cut into pieces for easier eating and blending of the melting cheeses. Spicy sausage, like chorizo, is a nice variation.

Fried Cheese Sticks

Perfect crust and gooey inside.

INGREDIENTS

8 ounces of mozzarella cheese cut into sticks, 1"x 1"
1 egg whisked for dipping
½ cup pork panko crumbs
animal fat: beef, lard, or bacon

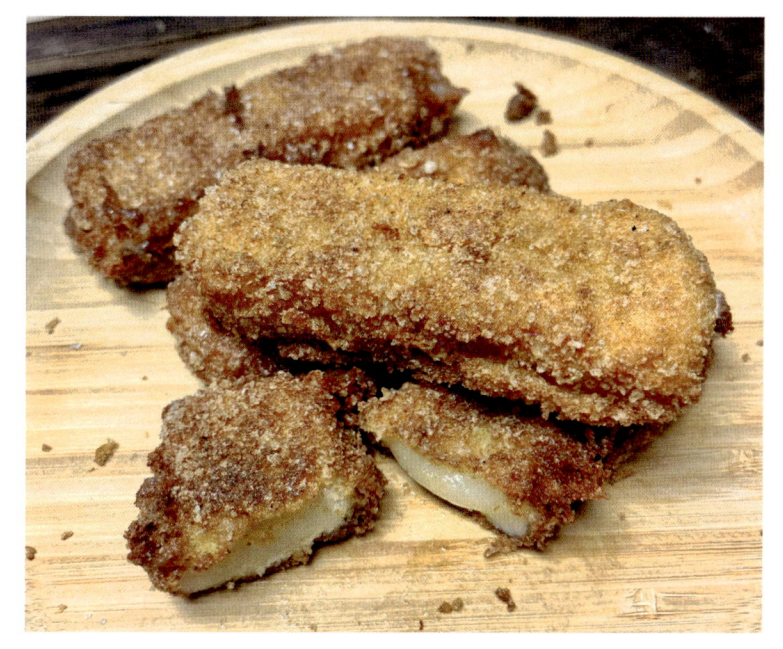

CARB COUNT: 6.5 GRAMS TOTAL

DIRECTIONS

Important: Freeze cheese at least 3 hours—after cutting into 1"x 1" thick sticks, before breading.

To cook, heat animal fat (lard or tallow works best) filled 1" deep in a skillet, set on medium to medium-high heat. Dip frozen cheese sticks in raw scrambled egg, then dip into the pork panko crumbs. Double coat them by dipping once again into the egg, followed by the pork panko yet again. Carefully lay cheese sticks into the popping hot grease. Cook on all sides for 1-2 minutes.

Notes: Do not overcook or the cheese will melt out. Smaller cut sticks also runs that risk. I use 8 ounces of Red Apple Cheese™ Apple Smoked Mozzarella, which cuts into 5 portions. Look for a block of cheese with good thickness. These have not been tested in an air fryer, though to enjoy the taste of pork fat in the crust, a brief bath in a grease-filled pan would be necessary before air frying for a few minutes. Deep frying might be the best solution.

Baked Burger Bun

This modified chaffle bun is sturdy and does not taste like eggs. It can also handle a ½-pound burger.

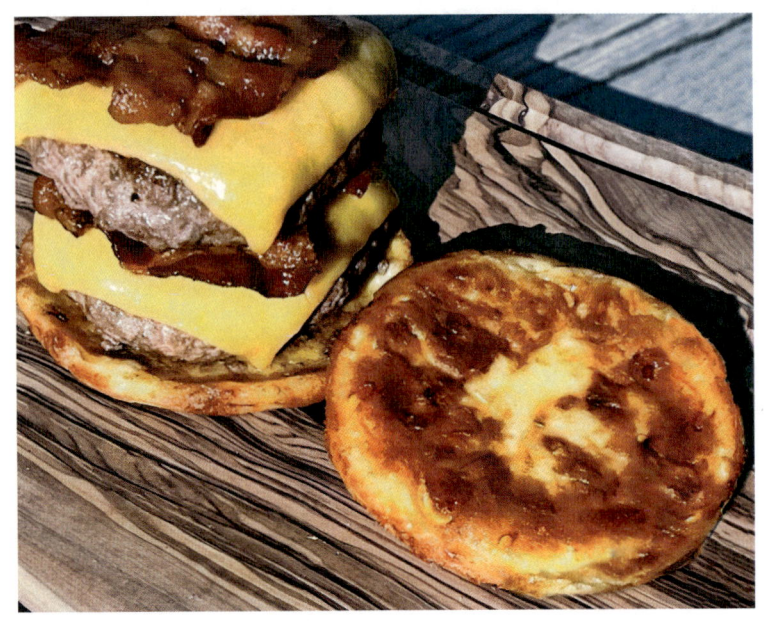

CARB COUNT: 2 GRAMS EACH

INGREDIENTS

2 eggs
1-2 cups mozzarella shreds
2 tablespoons marscapone
1 tablespoon gelatin
pinch of salt
butter to coat pans
optional:
garlic powder
onion powder

DIRECTIONS

Coat the bottom and sides of four 4" metal pie pans with butter, then set aside. Combine the other ingredients, starting by working the marscapone and eggs together before adding the shredded cheese. Sprinkle in the gelatin, and stir. Using an immersion blender, gets a smoother batter, especially if not using fine shredded cheese. Divide the batter evenly among the 4 pans, smoothing it flat. Bake at 365°F for about 15 minutes, then flip the buns over for an additional 5 minutes.

Notes: Buns can be baked in any shape, such as two 4"x 9" loaf pans for hoagie buns. If the buns stick, try lining pans with parchment paper and/or add more butter—or buy new. USA Pan makes a 3.5" multi-bun pan that is truly non-stick, or these 4" pans are available on Amazon in sets of 5.

Cheese Taco Shells

INGREDIENTS

1 cup (4 ½ ounces) shredded cheese, like cheddar, mozzarella, or a mix of both
parchment paper or silicone mat

Notes: You can use cheese slices to make these. Baking at a lower temperature makes them chewy.

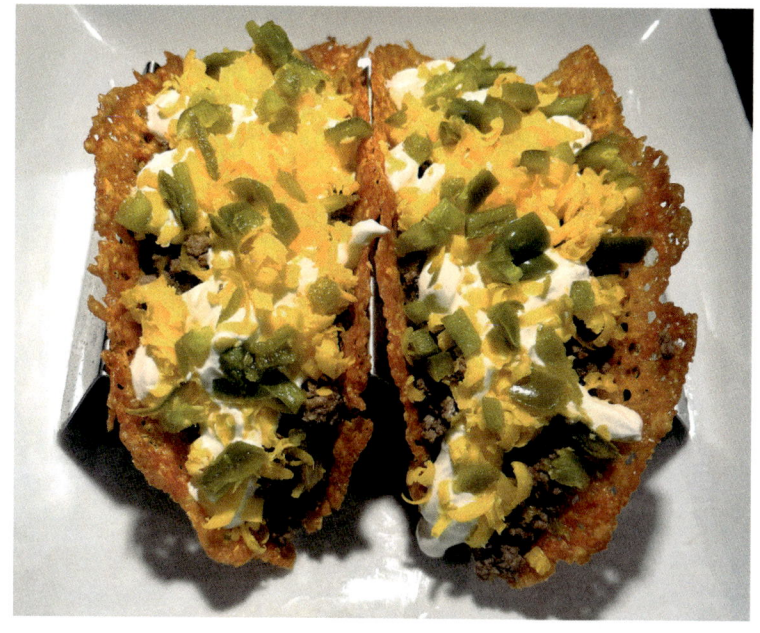

CARB COUNT: 1-2 GRAMS PER SHELL

DIRECTIONS

Set up your draping station by placing wide wooden cooking utensils balanced on top of jars. This will take some ingenuity if you don't have a taco shell rack. Preheat oven to 375°F. Line a large baking sheet with parchment paper. Portion out the shredded cheese as follows:
  Use ¼ cup (25-31 grams) of cheese to make 4 inch circles. This will yield 4 shells.
  Use ⅓ cup (1½ ounces or 40-45 grams) of cheese to make 5 inch circles. This will make 3 shells.
  Use ½ cup (60 grams) of cheese to make two 6 inch circles if you prefer them larger.

Bake for 7-10 minutes until completely melted and golden brown. Let them cool for a minute. Blot grease with a paper towel and then use a spatula to lift the circles and drape them over the long handles (or like a broom handle) that you should already have set up. Let the shells cool completely before removing and using. If you leave them flat, they can be used for tostadas, or to make cups, allow shells to firm up pressed down into muffin tins or draped over small bowls.

Extras

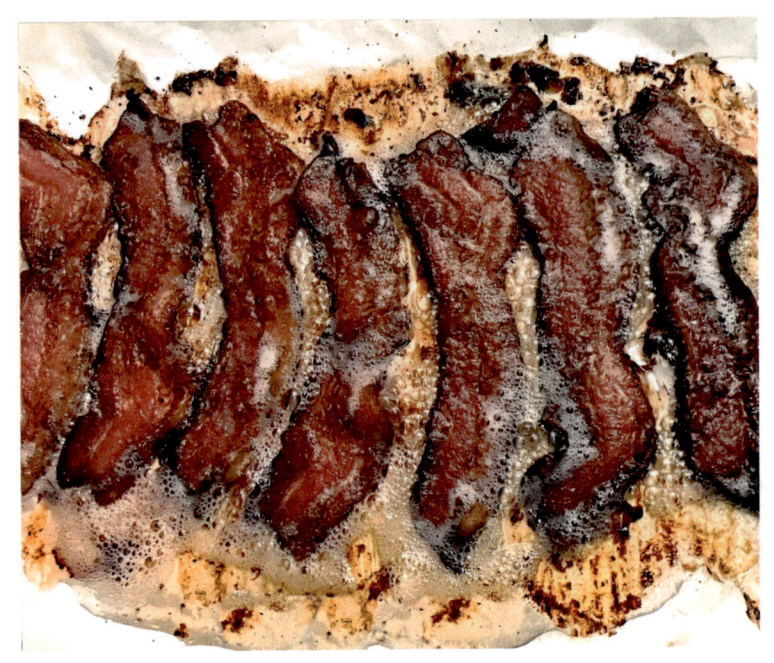

Oven Bacon

The easiest way to prepare large amounts of bacon at once

INGREDIENTS

bacon, thin or thick sliced
parchment paper

CARB COUNT: 0-2 GRAMS PER OUNCE

DIRECTIONS

Line a sheet pan with parchment paper, making sure it creates a sort of basket to contain the grease as the bacon cooks. This makes clean up super easy. Using a rack causes the bacon to stick to it, requiring soaking and scrubbing. Place bacon slices on the parchment, making sure they don't touch. Cook at 390° for 20-40 minutes depending on bacon thickness. At 20 minutes, check the bacon, and flip pieces over, rotating the pan for more even crisping.

Notes: Two half-sized sheet pans (13x18") will almost hold the fat double pack of Kirkland® bacon, leaving a few strips leftover. Two three-quarter-sized pans (15x21") are big enough, but hard to find. Full-sized sheet pans (18x26") are too big for most home ovens. Quarter-sized sheet pans (9.5x13") are very versatile, but the OXO® jellyroll pan (9x13") can even fit in the Breville® Smart Oven Air fryer Pro countertop toaster oven.

Bacon Onion Rings

Succulent and crispy

INGREDIENTS

12 ounces cold bacon, thin-sliced
2 medium onions cut into 1" rings

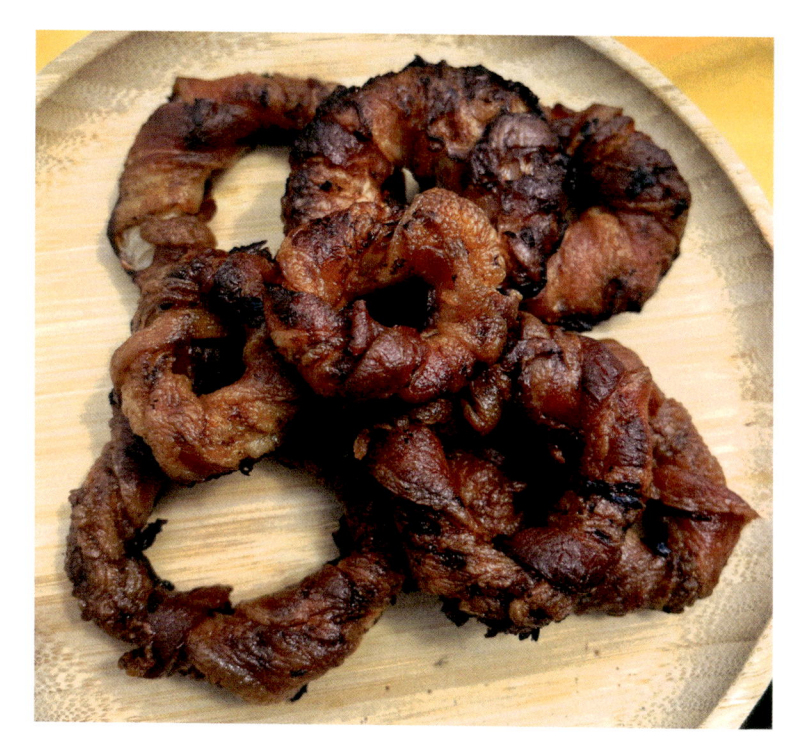

CARB COUNT: 3 GRAMS EACH

DIRECTIONS

Preheat oven to 350°F. Cut onions into 1" thick rings. When separating the rings, leave them doubled, or in other words use two rings to make one. Carefully and tightly wrap each ring with two pieces of bacon. Make sure to slightly overlap to account for shrinkage. Toothpicks broken in half can help to anchor the bacon if you need a third hand. Place assembled rings in a cast iron pan or a sheet tray lined with parchment. Bake them for about 15 minutes, before checking to see if they are ready to be flipped. Continue to check every 3-4 minutes, because they will all cook at different speeds due to being different sizes. When bacon is done to your liking, remove rings from the oven and drain on paper towels.

Note: These are worth the effort and can be easily re-heated in an air fryer if made ahead.

Pork Panko Breading Technique

This crunchy coating works for frying all kinds of meats.

INGREDIENTS

meat of choice
dry gelatin powder
seasonings of choice
whisked whole eggs
pork panko crumbs
tallow or lard for frying

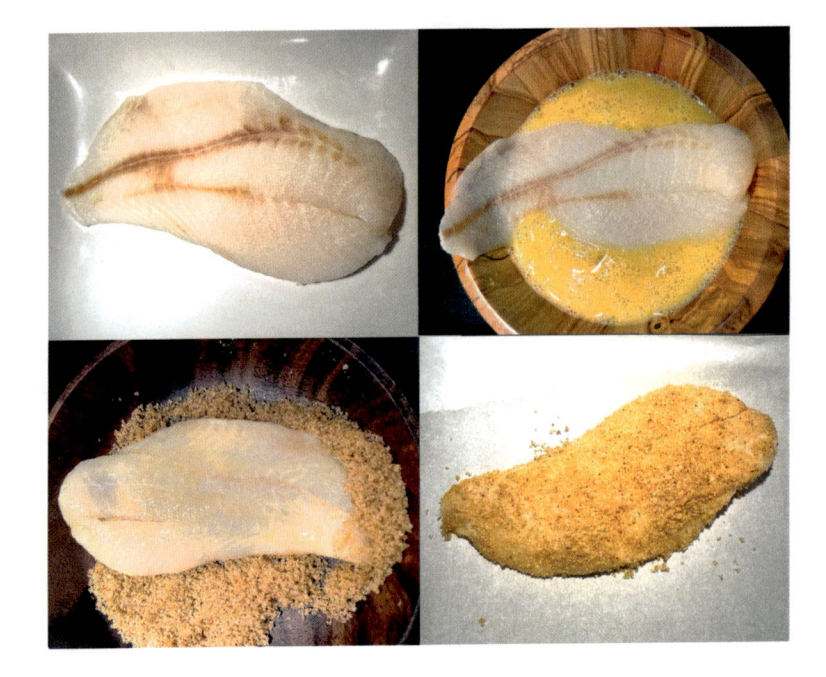

DIRECTIONS

This method works for shrimp, fish, chicken, beef, pork, venison, etc. Pat meat dry. You can season meat directly and then sprinkle lightly with gelatin powder. Keeping a shaker of it is very handy. The gelatin gives the egg more texture to cling to. Dip the meat into a bowl of whisked eggs, covering throughly. Shake off any extra. Keeping one hand wet for the eggs, and one hand dry to handle the meat in the crumb bowl, drop the egg-covered meat into the bowl set up with pork crumbs. You can also add seasoning to the panko if you like. Be sure to get good crumb coverage. Set breaded meat aside if you have multiple pieces to coat. Then proceed to fry in tallow or lard to the temperature your meat requires. Drain on a grate or paper towels before serving.

Notes: The texture of pork panko is more like course Japanese-style breadcrumbs, rather than traditional fine breadcrumbs. For other uses like retaining moisture and flavor, pork panko does not work very well compared to traditional bread.

Pork Rind Flatbread

Great alternative to chaffles, less firm, but also more like pita bread

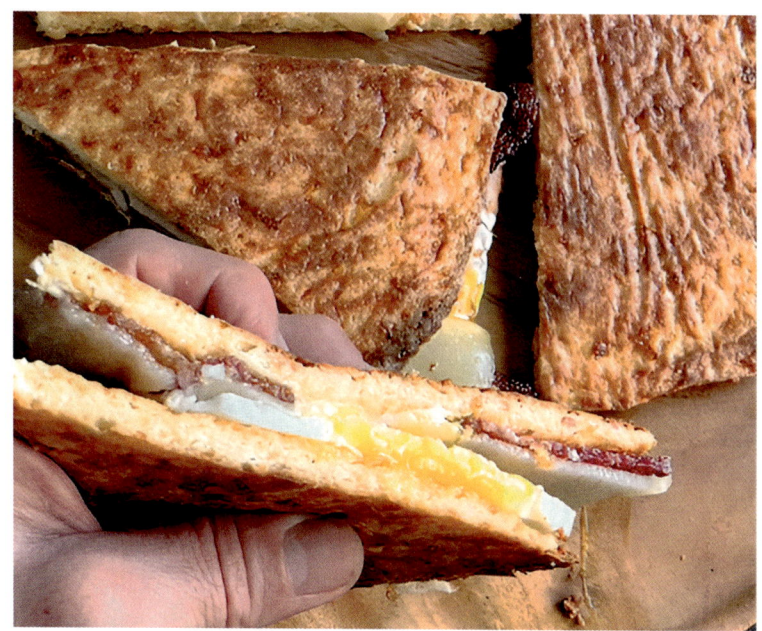

CARB COUNT: 18 GRAMS TOTAL

INGREDIENTS

1 ½ cups (115g) mozzarella shreds
8 ounces cream cheese, soft
3 eggs, room temperature
¾ cup (30g) pork panko crumbs

DIRECTIONS

Allow ingredients to come to room temperature. Shred the mozzarella. Use an immersion blender to incorporate the eggs into the cream cheese, adding the shredded cheese, and then the pork crumbs. Preheat oven to 375°F.

Using two pieces of parchment, flatten the dough out into the shape you want—round, square, or rectangular—using a rolling pin if you have one, a flat bottom pan, or even your hands. Aim for a thickness of 1 cm. Remove the top parchment sheet and lift the dough onto a baking sheet. Bake for 20-25 minutes. Cut into smaller shapes as desired.

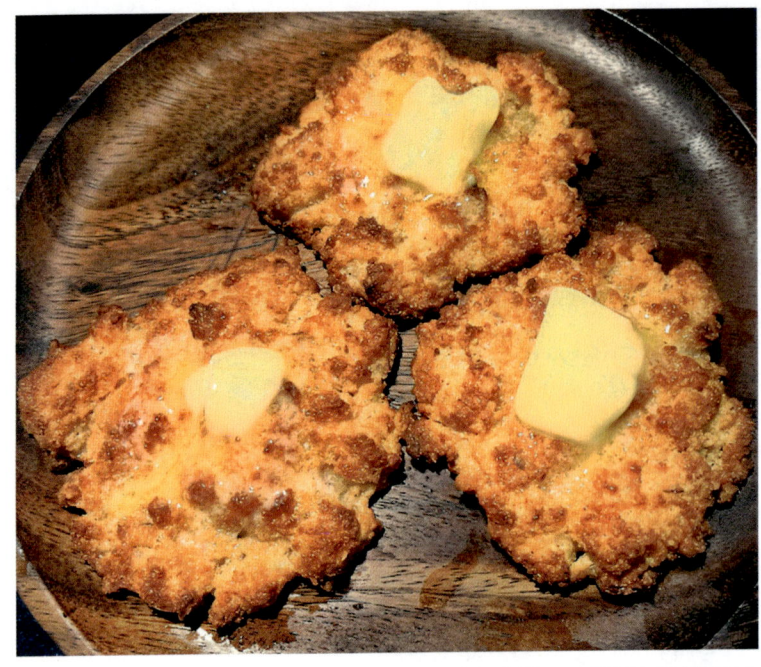

Friscuits

Pork rind cheddar biscuits

CARB COUNT: 3.7 GRAMS TOTAL

INGREDIENTS

1 egg
¾ cup (30g) pork panko crumbs
¾ cup (28g) shredded cheese
1 tablespoon sour cream
1 tablespoon grated Parmesan
½ teaspoon baking powder
pinch of salt

DIRECTIONS

Prepare the pork rinds into course crumbs in a food processor. Whisk the egg with the sour cream before combing all ingredients in a bowl. Stir to bring it all together. Divide batter into 3 or 4 portions with a spoon or a disher. Place on a sheet pan lined with parchment paper. Bake at 450°F for 12 minutes. Makes 3-4 biscuits.

Notes: It's easy to turn these into herb biscuits by adding ¼ teaspoon garlic powder, and/or combinations of rosemary, chives, sage, dill, parsley, or thyme. Dried herbs work, but fresh are transformative with their aromas.

Pork Rind Stuffing

Double or triple this for company.

INGREDIENTS

¼ cup minced celery
¼ cup minced onion
2 tablespoons butter
3 ¼ oz (90g) ground pork rinds
2 eggs
½ cup chicken stock
1 tablespoon fresh thyme
1 tablespoon fresh rosemary

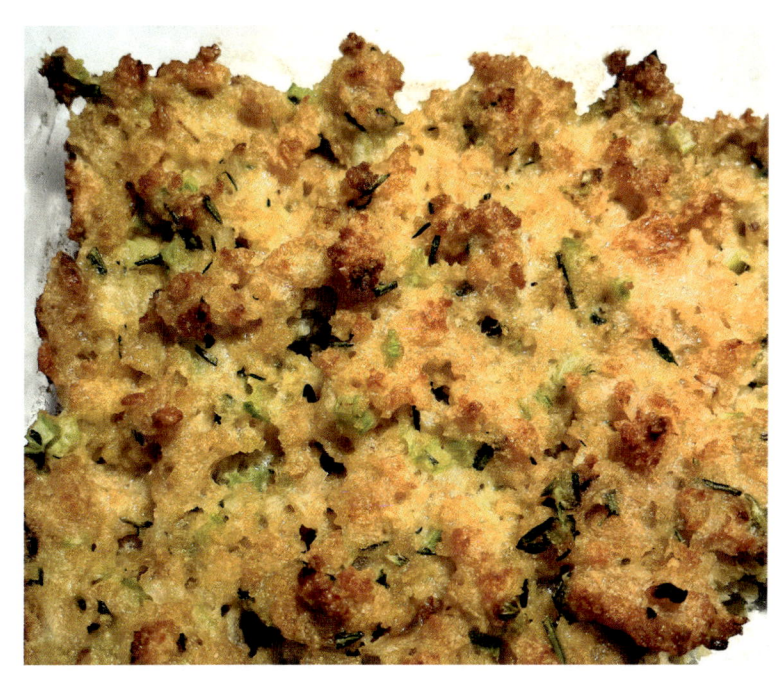

CARB COUNT: 5 GRAMS TOTAL

DIRECTIONS

Sauté celery and onion in melted butter until soft. Grind the pork rinds in a food processor until pieces are pebble-sized and smaller. Do not use the darker and harder pieces as they will end up chewy. Combine all ingredients and mix thoroughly. The amount of stock needed varies with how finely ground the crumbs are. The mixture should be moist enough to form crumbly cakes. Pack loosely though, and bake at 400°F in a Pyrex baking pan for 20-25 minutes. The pan pictured here is 7.25" x 5.5". Makes 2 servings. If you want it crispy and crunchy, fry it up in a skillet.

Notes: Makes 2 servings. A 3.25 oz bag of pork rinds = 2 cups of pork rind crumbs. The amount of stock you need varies according to how finely you grind the pork rind crumbs. The mixture should be wet enough to form crumbly cakes if you were to pack them. Use the best tasting, un-flavored pork rinds you can find. The fresh rosemary and thyme really complete the dish. Dried herbs will work though. Goes great with my reduction gravy recipe on page 66.

Cauliflower Mash

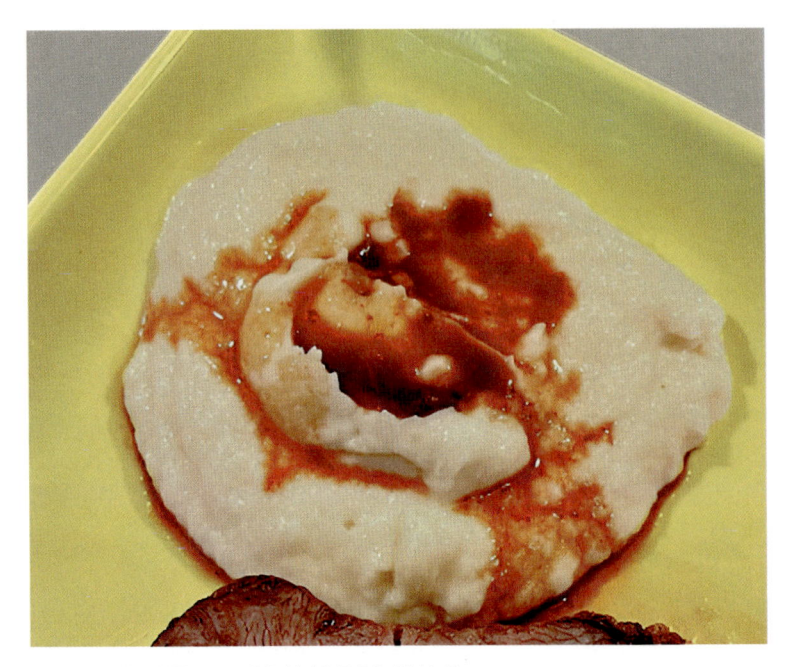

Delicious by itself, or use it for reverse Shepard's pie

CARB COUNT: 12.3 GRAMS FOR HALF

INGREDIENTS

13 cups (500g) cauliflower
2 tablespoons heavy cream
½ teaspoon garlic powder
½ cup shredded white cheese
2 ounces crème fraîche, goat cheese, or cream cheese

DIRECTIONS

Chop up the cauliflower then boil for 12 minutes, or until soft. Pour into a colander to drain, and let the steam evaporate. Use a food processor to blend all of the ingredients until smooth. Should yield 2 fat portions.

Notes: For a reverse shepherd's pie, top the cauliflower mash with 1½ pounds browned 85% ground beef, and pour a batch and a half of reduction gravy over it all. You can add cheese too.

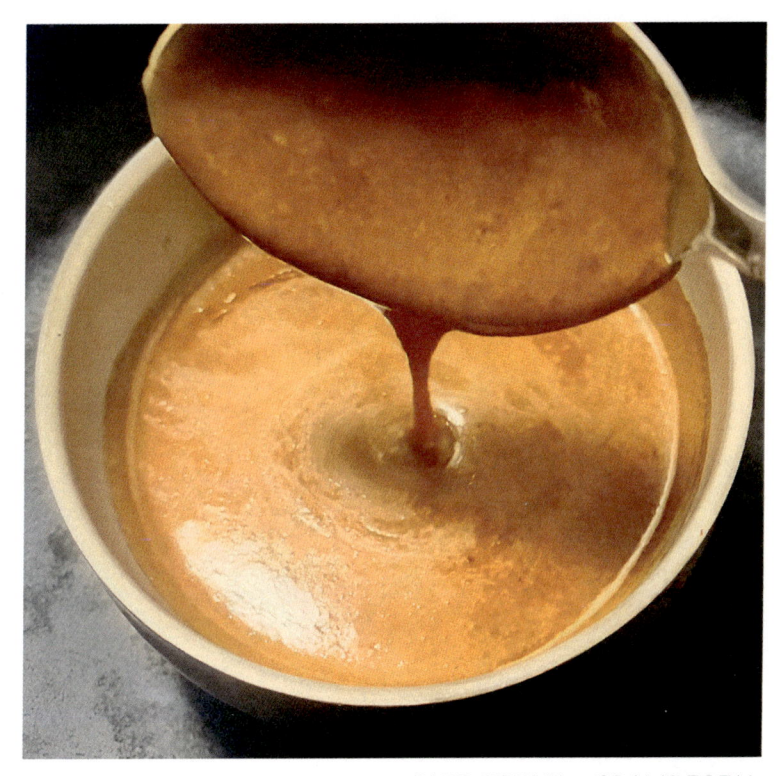

No-Flour Reduction Gravy

Simple yet rich and delicious

CARB COUNT: 7 GRAMS TOTAL

INGREDIENTS

2 cups (473 ml) stock
1 cup (236 ml) heavy cream
garlic powder (optional)
onion powder (optional)

DIRECTIONS

Add all ingredients to a skillet or a saucepan. Cook down the liquid by using medium-high heat for about 20 minutes or until desired thickness is achieved. Stir frequently. Only add salt after it has finished reducing. The salt in the stock will intensify as the sauce concentrates.

Notes: Works with any kind of stock. Fatty drippings may cause separation issues. Using a broth or stock with minimal fat gets the best results. Yields 3/4 cup once reduced.

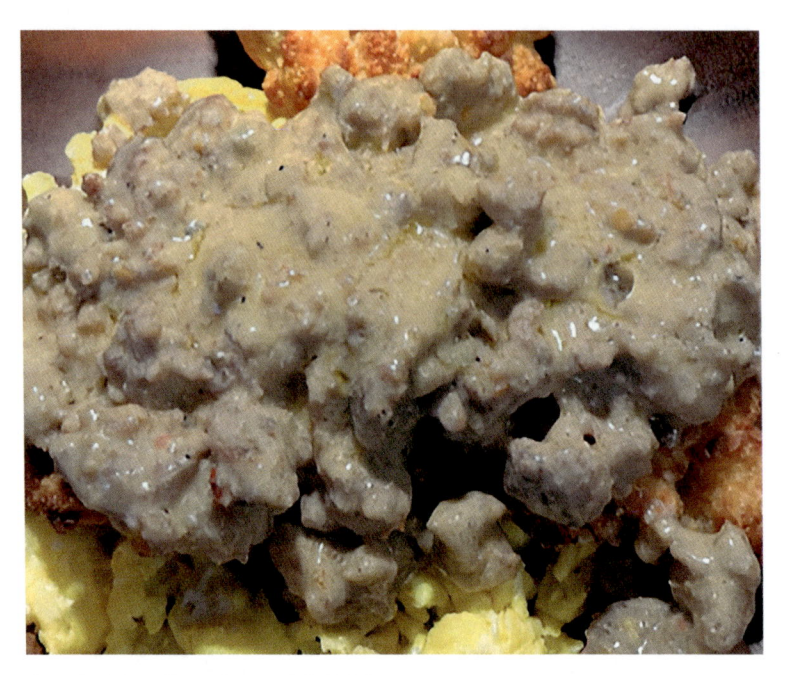

Flourless Sausage Gravy

Good with plain ground pork, or with seasoned sausage.

CARB COUNT: 8 GRAMS TOTAL

INGREDIENTS

1 pound ground sausage
2 cups stock, beef or chicken
1 cup heavy cream
salt & pepper

DIRECTIONS

Brown the sausage in a skillet. Drain as much grease off as you can or it may affect the emulsion of the gravy. Pour both the stock and the cream into the skillet and simmer to thicken the sauce until it is reduced to gravy consistency. This should take about 15-20 minutes over medium-high heat. If it looks too oily, add more cream until it looks right. Add seasonings to taste.

Simple White Alfredo Sauce

A rich and creamy sauce that can be used for dressing up dishes

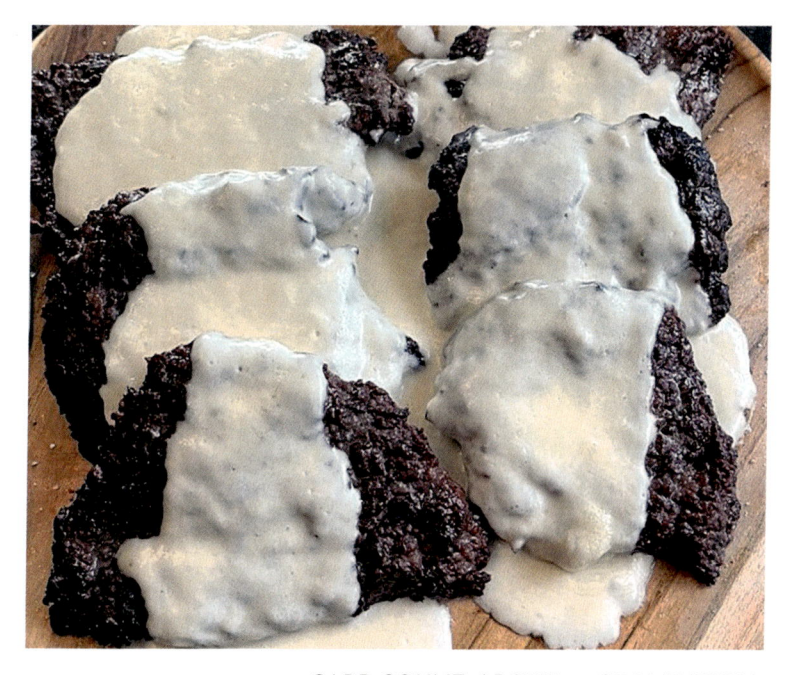

CARB COUNT: ABOUT 27 GRAMS TOTAL

INGREDIENTS

2 cups heavy cream
¾-1 cup fresh Parmesan cheese
1-4 tablespoons butter
pinch of nutmeg (optional)
garlic powder (optional)
4 ounces cream cheese (optional)

DIRECTIONS

In a small sauce pan, bring cream and butter to a quick boil. Turn down the heat, add the cheese using a whisk. Barely simmer over low heat until desired thickness is achieved. It's important not to overheat your sauce. Melted cheese will break and separate once it gets too hot. Turn heat off and sauce will thicken further. If you need a truly thick sauce, add some cream cheese to give more body.

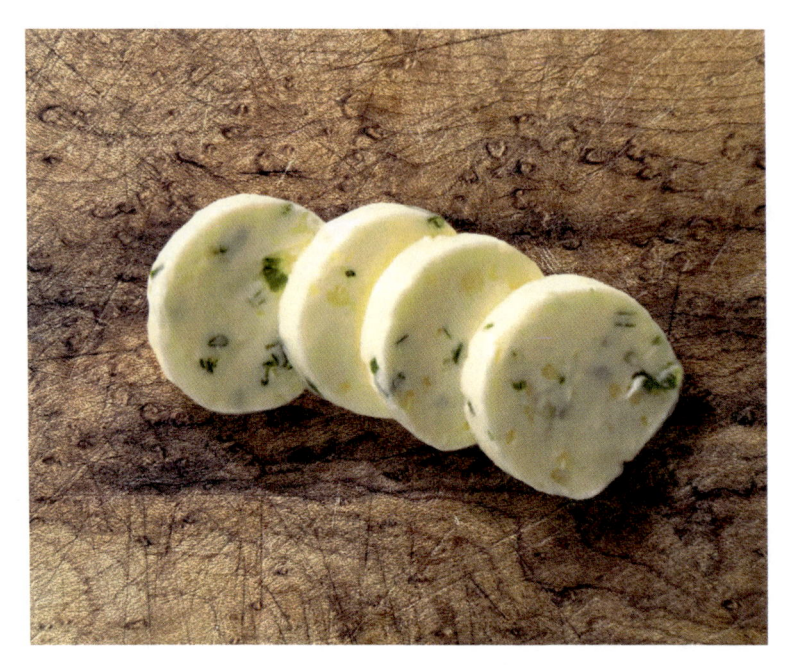

Goat Cheese-Chive Butter

CARB COUNT: 5.6 GRAMS TOTAL

INGREDIENTS

2 sticks salted butter
4 ounces goat cheese
⅓ cup chives or green onions
2 tablespoon fresh garlic
salt to taste

DIRECTIONS

Be sure to let the butter and cheese come to room temperature so they are soft enough to work with. Mince up the garlic and chives. (Herb scissors are great here.) In a bowl, combine all ingredients using the whisk attachment on an immersion blender if you have one, or do it by hand. Once it comes together, spread it onto parchment or waxed paper in a log shape, then roll it up and freeze. Cut portions off as needed.

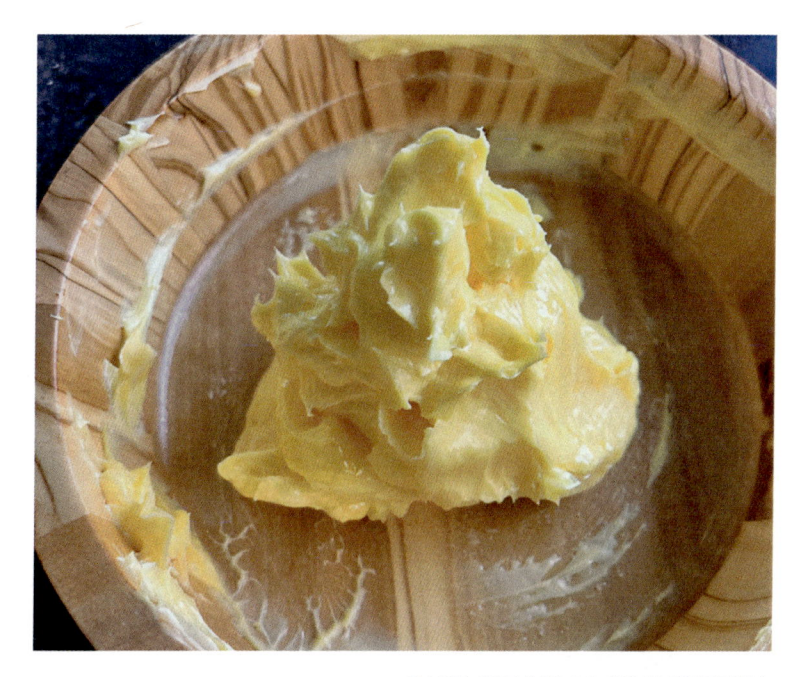

Butter Mayo

Almost like Hollandaise, but just the basics, and raw. This can be used as a base for other things.

CARB COUNT: 1.5 GRAMS TOTAL

INGREDIENTS

3 egg yolks
6 tablespoons (85g) soft butter

DIRECTIONS

Let eggs and butter come to room temperature. Use an immersion blender to combine egg yolks and butter. The consistency you end up with is determined by how soft your butter is. Barely soft gets the best mayo-like result, though barely melted works also.

Notes: This is raw. If you have a health concern, use pasteurized eggs, or whisk yolks in a pan and melt the butter, taking the temperature up to 160°F, which is about when the a spoon will remain coated with a film. This is a great mayo replacement and makes a flexible base for many sauces. The concept of butter mayo comes from @MariaEmmerich on X, who uses lemon juice and Dijon in her version.

Low CarBBQ Sauce

INGREDIENTS

2 tablespoons butter
1 cup stevia sweetened ketchup
1 ½ tablespoon Worcestershire
1 tablespoon hot sauce
½ tablespoon apple cider vinegar
½ teaspoon garlic powder
½ teaspoon onion powder
½ teaspoon unsweetened cocoa
½ teaspoon salt
¼ teaspoon cumin
¼ teaspoon paprika
¼ teaspoon chili powder
⅛ teaspoon cayenne pepper

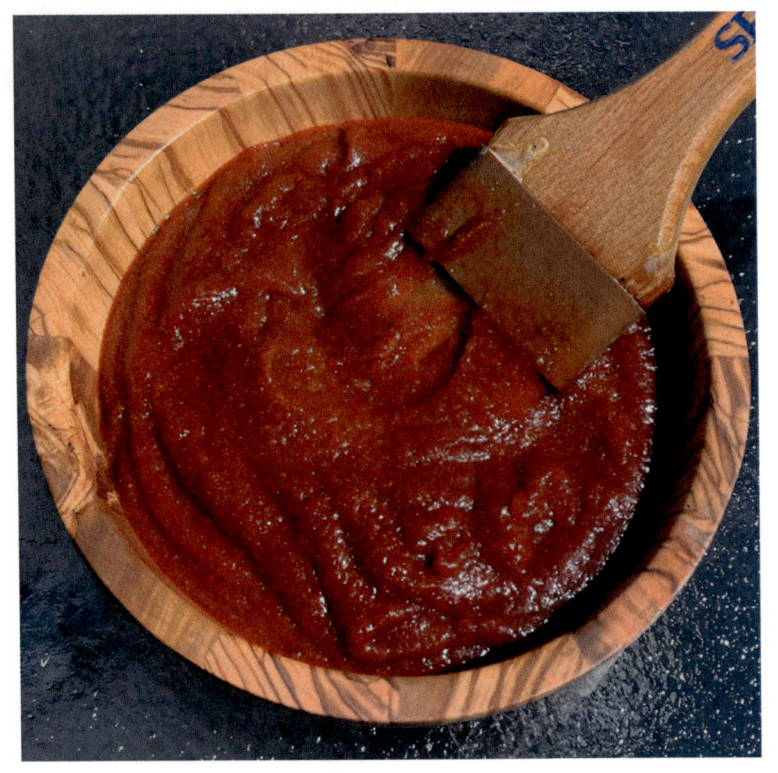

CARB COUNT: 39 GRAMS TOTAL or 2 GRAMS PER TABLESPOON

DIRECTIONS

Melt butter and add all ingredients. Stir until combined on low heat to let the flavors marry. Feel free to make it sweeter.

Notes: Primal® unsweetened ketchup makes a good base, or French's® with stevia. This can be made without a lot of heat. Adjust the amounts for personal taste.
For sweetening, Besti® Brown Monk Fruit Sweetener with Allulose is a natural carb-free sweetener that will caramelize. It has a slight maple flavor, and replaces brown sugar. Molasses, maple syrup, or honey may also be used to sweeten the sauce.

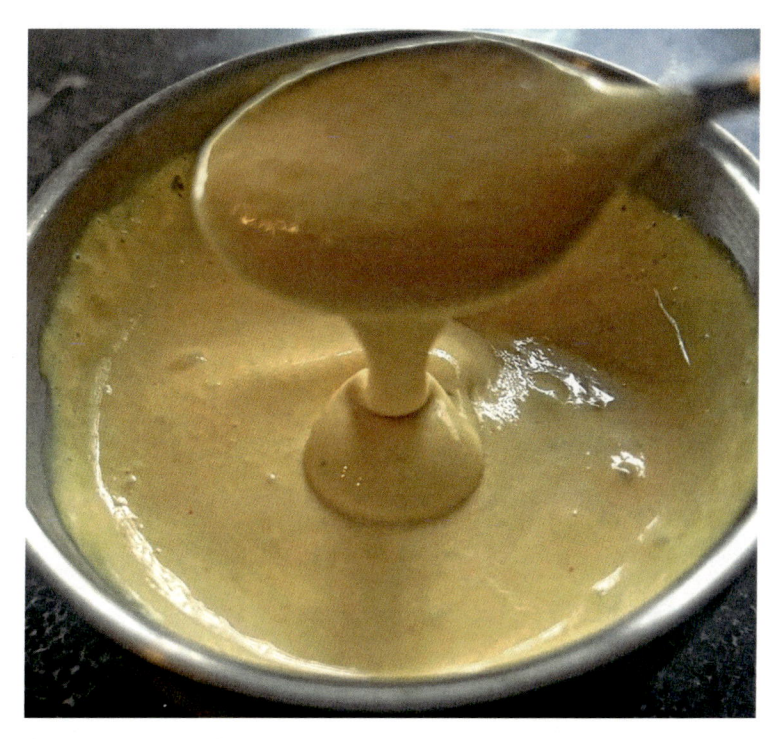

Keto "Big Mac®" Sauce

CARB COUNT: 8 GRAMS

INGREDIENTS

¼ cup melted butter
3 egg yolks
1 tablespoon dill pickles, chopped
3+ tablespoon no-sugar ketchup
garlic and onion powder
pinch of salt

DIRECTIONS

Melt the butter, then combine with the egg yolks using an immersion blender. Roughly chop the pickles. Add all the ingredients, starting with a few shakes of garlic and onion powders and blend again. Adjust the seasonings to taste. Refrigerate for at least 30 minutes to thicken.

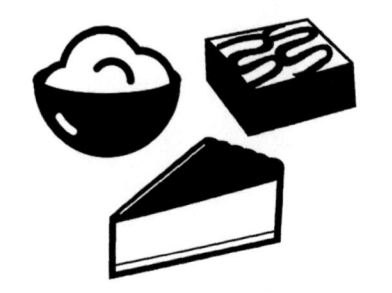

Desserts

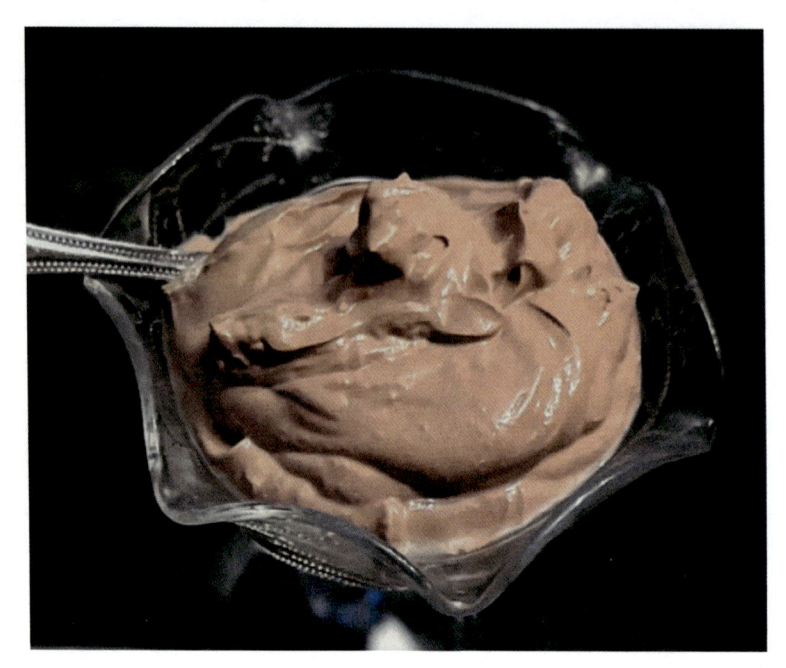

Whipped Cocoa Yogurt

CARB COUNT: 12 GRAMS

INGREDIENTS

1 cup Greek yogurt
½ cup heavy cream
1 tablespoon cocoa powder
optional: bit of allulose or honey

DIRECTIONS

This is a quick dessert snack. Simply put the ingredients together in a bowl and use an immersion blender to combine them until smooth. For some sweetness, a few pinches of allulose will do the trick.

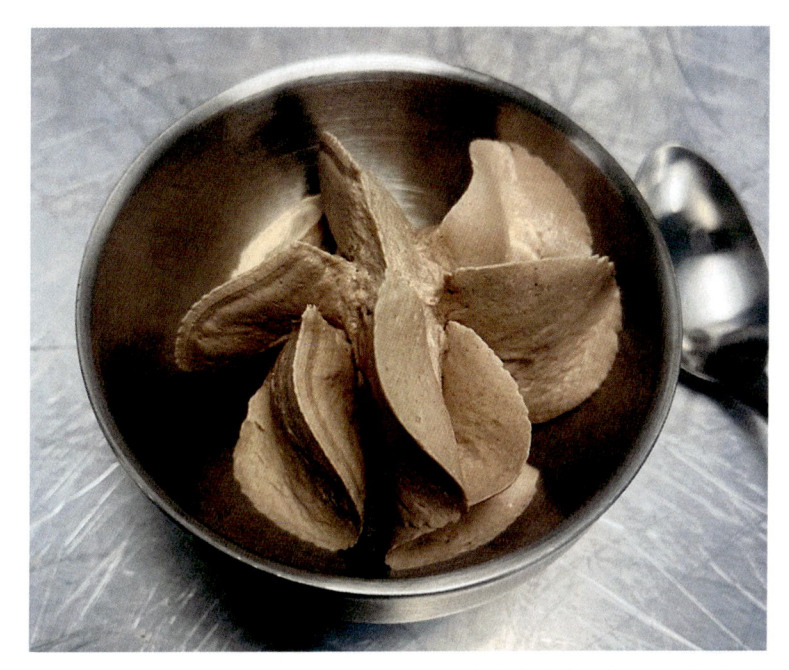

Keto Chocolate Mousse

CARB COUNT: 10.2 GRAMS

INGREDIENTS

½ cup (100g) soft cream cheese
½ cup (118 ml) heavy cream
1 tablespoon unsweetened cocoa
splash of vanilla extract
optional: a pinch of sweetener

DIRECTIONS

Start with room-temperature ingredients so the cream cheese is soft and pliable, and the heavy cream won't make it stiffen up when combined. Blend the cocoa and vanilla into the cream to dissolve first. Then blend all ingredients with an immersion blender for about 30 seconds.

Note: Greek yogurt can be substituted for cream cheese.

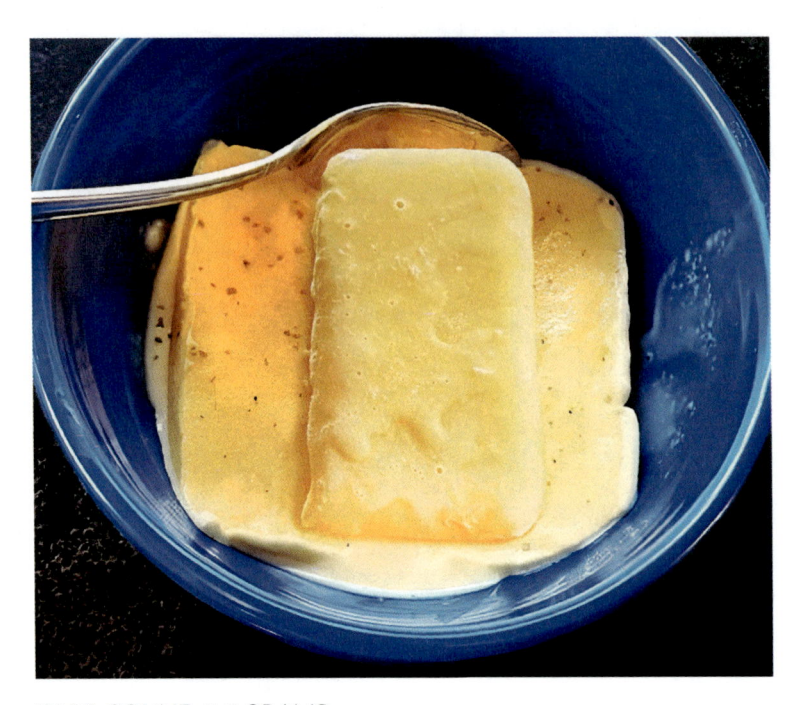

Vanilla Custard Ice Cream

This is my most viewed recipe online

CARB COUNT: 11.7 GRAMS

INGREDIENTS

1 ½ cups (354 ml) heavy cream
3 egg yolks
1 tablespoon vanilla extract
4 tablespoons (50g) allulose

DIRECTIONS

Add the cream and 3 egg yolks to a small saucepan. Heat gently but don't boil, while stirring to scrape the bottom of the pan, about 5 minutes. When the spatula stays slightly coated, the eggs are thickened. Add the extract, and sweetener or salt, to taste before pouring in a shallow pan to freeze. This can also be churned in an ice cream maker.

Notes: Once frozen it will taste less sweet. 2 tablespoons (30g) cocoa powder can be added for chocolate flavor. Extracts such as maple, lemon, orange, coconut, or mint expand the possibilities. So do instant coffee, a bit of salt, or add-ins like fruit or chocolate chips.

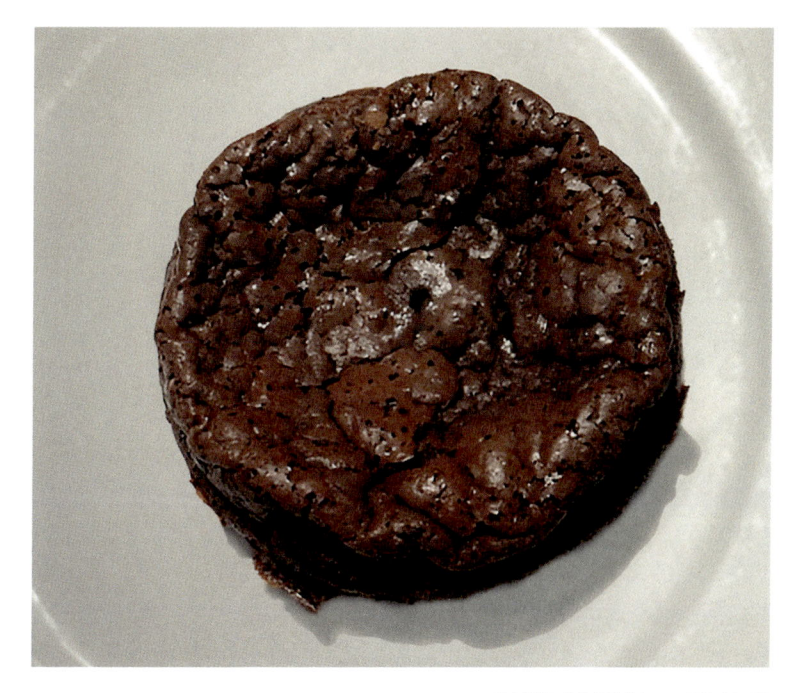

No-Flour Brownie

Tastes just like a brownie should

CARB COUNT: 13 GRAMS

INGREDIENTS

1 egg
½ or 1 teaspoon vanilla extract
2 tablespoons soft cream cheese
1 ½ tablespoons cocoa powder
2 tablespoons allulose sweetener

½ tablespoon melted butter

DIRECTIONS

Bring cream cheese and egg to room-temperature. Mix the unsweetened cocoa powder with the allulose first to work out clumps. Use a mixer, immersion blender, or mini food processor to combine ingredients. Pour the butter in a small pie pan, 4" ramekin, or mini spring-form pan to grease the bottom. If you have parchment paper, you can line the pan to avoid sticking. Bake at 350°F for about 20 minutes.

Notes: A pinch of espresso powder will boost the flavor. While this recipe can be scaled up, it really is nicer in smaller portions for the crispy edges. Beware that it doubles in volume while baking before deflating, so choose your pan carefully.

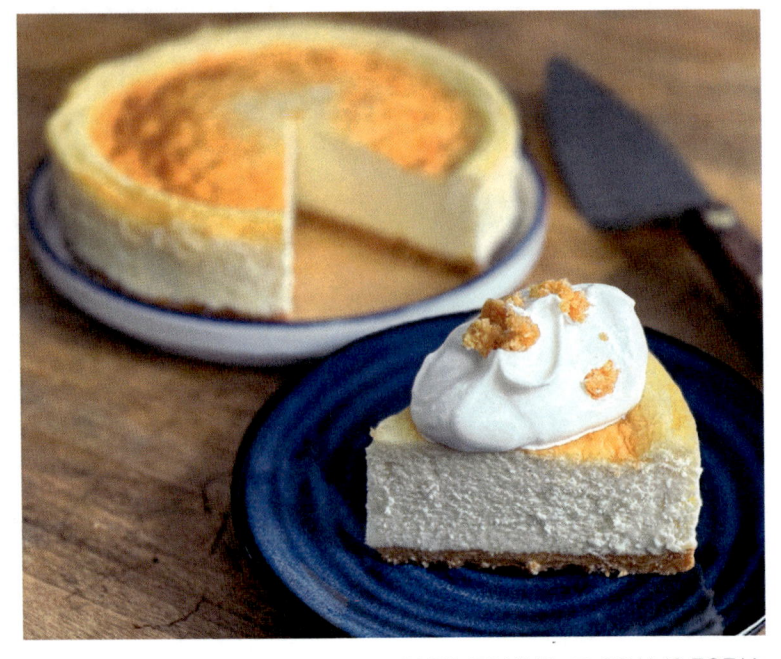

Carnivore Cheesecake

Caramelized non-fat milk substitutes for a graham cracker crust

CARB COUNT: 63 GRAMS TOTAL

INGREDIENTS

Crumble crust:
4-6 tablespoons salted butter
½ cup (65g) nonfat milk powder

Batter:
8 ounces cream cheese, soft
8 ounces mascarpone, soft
4 teaspoons vanilla extract
2-4 tablespoons allulose
3 eggs, room temperature
zest from 1 lemon, optional

Topping:
½ cup heavy cream, chilled
2 tablespoons mascarpone
1 tablespoon vanilla
1 tablespoon allulose

Pan Options:
round springform pans: 7", 8," or 9"(will be thin)
small round pans: 5"(x2), 4"(x3), 3"(x4)
square pans: 6", 7," or 8"
rectangle pans: 6"x9" or 8"x4" loaf

DIRECTIONS

Make the crust by first caramelizing the milk powder in a skillet. Over medium-low heat, melt a the salted butter. Sprinkle the half cup of milk powder over the butter in the pan. Add more powdered milk if it looks like there's too much butter. Stir frequently as it is browning. This may take about 20 minutes.

Once the dry milk is sufficiently caramelized, spread the "wet sand" into the bottom of your pan of choice, like ramekins, or a 7" or 8" spring-form pan lined with a circle of parchment paper. If your pan leaks and you want to use the water bath method, wrap foil around the outside of the pan—or just use a regular cake pan. It is not necessary to press the crumbles flat because the butter causes it to settle. Set aside.

Make the batter. Add the cheeses to a mixing bowl along with the vanilla and the sweetener. Use a mixer to cream the room temperature ingredients together. Add the eggs one at a time, mixing between additions. Adjust sweetness to taste. Pour the liquid batter into the prepared cake pan.

Preheat your oven to 325°F and prepare your moat—if using. Place the cake pan inside a slightly larger cake pan. Boil a few cups of water, and pour the hot water into the larger outer pan so that the water surrounds the cake, and comes half way up the sides of it. This will help the cheesecake to bake more evenly and slowly for a creamier texture. Pouring the water once the pans are on the middle rack in the oven may help prevent a spill. Bake for *about* 1 hour and 10 minutes, and *if not using a water-bath, bake at 300°F for about 50-60 minutes instead.* Pan sizes will change bake times, so keep an eye on the oven. Ramekins will take about 25 to bake at 300°F.

Check doneness by how wiggly the very center of the cake is. It should not be liquidy. The edges should be firm, and the very center should still have a little jiggle to it. The cake will continue to cook as it cools. Prop the door open and let the cake rest in the oven 20-30 minutes. Then remove the cake pan from the oven and water bath to a cooling rack. Allow the cake to cool about 1-2 hours before chilling it for 6 hours or overnight—only if you want the best texture. It's great without the fuss too!

Prepare the topping. Use cold ingredients here. Whip the heavy cream with the mascarpone, vanilla, and sweetener until fluffy. This takes about two minutes. Serve with whipped topping and any extra crumbles. enjoy!

Index

Meat Dishes 2
Dry Brining 3
Picanha Roast 5
Chateaubriand 6
Brisket, Slow-Cooked & Instant Pot 7
Instant Pot Skewered Brisket 8
Easy Chuck Roast Soup 9
Crockpot Roast 10
Spicy Mongolian Beef 11
Bulgogi Marinade 12
Oven Ribs 13
Next-Level Short Ribs 15
Korean BBQ Short Ribs 16
Sloppy Joes 17
Meat-Lovers Chuck Eye Chili 18
Bolognese 19
Meatloaf 20
Hamburger Hash 21
Enchilada Dip 22
Jalapeño Popper Cheese-Steak 23
Jalapeno Popper Pork Chop 24
Smoked Brisket 25
Smoked Kabobs 26
Smoked Oxtails 27
Smoked Meatballs 28